DIET RIGHT!

DIET RIGHT!

The Consumer's Guide to Diet and Weight Loss Programs

By Matthew Quincy
Foreword by Mary K. Young, M.S., R.D.

Conari Press
Berkeley, CA

Copyright © 1991 by Matthew Quincy
Foreword copyright © 1991 by Mary K. Young

Printed in the United States of America

Cover by Robert Steven Pawlak Design

ISBN: 0-943233-10-0

LCC: 90-846371

Table of Contents

Foreword

Weight is a serious problem in the United States. Approximately 80 million Americans are overweight; half of those are considered to be obese and 11 million are considered severely obese. According to the Department of Health and Human Services, the average man is 18 pounds overweight and the average woman is 21 pounds overweight. Between the ages of 25 and 50, the typical American gradually gains between 15 and 20 pounds.

But the problem is not limited to adults. The incidence of obesity in children and adolescents has increased by more than 50 percent in the last two decades and more than ten million schoolchildren in the U.S. are now considered overweight.

These figures are cause for concern because obesity is associated with numerous health problems such as high blood pressure, coronary artery disease, abnormally high levels of blood fats (cholesterol, triglycerides), and adult-onset diabetes. Obese people are more likely to suffer from muscular and skeletal problems, respiratory difficulties, and surgical complications. Obese men have an increased risk of developing cancers of the colon, rectum, and prostate while obese women have a greater chance of suffering from cancers of the gall bladder, bile passages, breast, cervix, uterus, and ovaries.

Being overweight can also cause psychological problems. An obese person generally suffers from low self esteem, is anxious and depressed. He or she may experience economic and social discrimination as well. Our society is thin oriented and we reward those who fit in. Therefore overweight people may be social outcasts, receive lower salaries than thin colleagues, and pay higher insurance premiums.

In search of a miraculous solution to weight problems, many of us have tried everything and anything– with little success. Most methods have proved fruitless; some are potentially dangerous. We often end up in worse shape with more weight and fat to lose than we started with.

So what's the answer? From a scientific standpoint, it is uncomplicated. Weight maintenance involves an equilibrium between calories consumed and calories burned. Therefore, the number of calories you consume and your level of physical activity will determine if you maintain, gain, or lose weight. This sounds simple, but in practice, it proves quite difficult for many people to control, as evidenced by the vast number of overweight people in the United States and the enormous number of fad diets and weight loss programs available.

To succeed in the long run requires four things: responsibility, commitment, a sound plan, and behavior modification. First, you must take responsibility for your weight problem and stop blaming something or someone else. You must also be committed to your goal. You should consume a well-balanced, nutritious diet in appropriate amounts, and exercise regularly. Lastly, you need to address negative food and exercise behaviors that hinder your ability to succeed. We all become overweight for reasons. If these are not addressed and dealt with, I can guarantee you will eventually regain the weight you previously lost.

This is not to say that organized programs or diets are not beneficial. They certainly can be, given that the program is well matched to an individual's personal requirements. This is important because, just as we all have different eye and hair color, personalities, and body shape, we also differ in the best method to solve weight problems and achieve success.

It is my hope that this book will provide the necessary information you require to make an informed choice as to which program or diet best fits your personal needs. But as you peruse the material, remember a good program will adequately address good nutrition and negative behaviors, and provide for exercise. Most of all, you must take responsibility and be committed.

Good luck and much success!

Mary K. Young, M.S. R.D.
Registered Dietitian at the
University of Chicago Hospitals

A Brief Word About this Book

I undertook this project in the belief that those in search of a helping hand to deal with their weight problems could benefit from a resource that laid open the options in as much detail and with as much unbiased information as possible. All too often the weight loss industry advertises and promotes itself solely on the basis of celebrity endorsements and testimonials. But what works for one person is not necessarily a good program for another, or more importantly, not a particularly good basis upon which to make a decision.

I have attempted to provide a helpful overview of the major diet and weight loss programs available, but at times, doing the research for this book was frustrating. Getting the information to compile this book was complicated by a high degree of fear and suspicion prevalent within some quarters of the industry. The diet industry has grown to enormous proportions and with that growth considerable dollars (over $30 billion is spent yearly in the United States on diet related products and services) is now at stake.

As a whole, the industry is composed of many people truly dedicated to helping overweight people achieve lasting, healthy weight loss. But like any other pursuit there are those involved who are strictly there to make a fast buck. Recently the U.S. Senate held a number of hearings concerning the safety, effectiveness, and marketing approaches of those within the industry. Pressure is mounting for the Food and Drug Administration (FDA) to take a more aggressive stance in dealing with diet-related products, and just recently the FDA announced its intention to ban 111 ingredients in non-prescription diet drug products. Responding to that pressure, the Federal Trade Commission has pledged to take a more active role in policing the advertising practices of weight loss businesses. Additionally, a number of lawsuits have been filed across the country against a number of programs, alleging unsafe practices and lack of warnings, and resulting physical injuries.

As a result, my request for detailed information about how different programs operate was sometimes met with suspicion, at times hampered by a lack of cooperation and on two occasions was met with a flat refusal to respond. It should be noted, however, that for the most part the people within the industry were professional, helpful and even enthusiastic about the potential of a guide of this nature.

In selecting the programs to include, I attempted to include every program large enough to have an impact in the marketplace. Some programs operate internationally, others are nationwide chains; still others are restricted to particular states. Even though every reader will not have access to all the programs listed, it is often the smaller program that offers the more innovative approaches, and so I felt that their inclusion in the book was appropriate.

The information contained in the listings was drawn from materials acquired from the programs themselves as well as interviews with principals within the organizations. I have attempted to be as descriptive and informative as possible. Obviously the prices quoted in the book are, of necessity, estimates. Prices change regularly; special offers are common. Different locations cost more or less depending on the local cost of living, rent, etc.; and people with differing amounts of weight to lose may pay more or less depending on their situation. So use the price information as a general guideline in comparing the costs of different programs, but make sure to double check prices and possible availability of seasonal specials before committing to any particular program.

5

Additionally, the weight loss industry is a highly competitive one. While the information gathered for this book was current at the time the book was published, I did find that programs react to a changing market with incredible speed and the exact particulars of any given program may change. I would suggest double checking with programs that sound interesting to you before signing up and make sure the features of the program that attracted you in the first place are still being offered.

The listings in this book are organized into five general categories:

Moderate Calorie/Grocery Store Food Programs: These programs are designed to assist you in making the proper food choices for a healthy diet and rely on your ability to prepare meals from grocery store food with menu assistance.

Packaged Food Programs: With these plans your diet consists of packaged, calorie-controlled foods that you purchase through the particular program.

Very Low Calorie Diets: With these systems you completely replace your regular diet with special formulated low calorie/high nutritional value products, and participate in a program of close physician monitoring.

Combination Programs: These offer some mixture of grocery store food and Very Low Calorie Diet supplements.

Other Weight Loss Approaches: This category is a catchall for those programs that do not fit neatly into one of the categories above.

We intend to update this guide on a regular basis in order to keep up with the rapid changes within the industry. Your help would be appreciated. If your experience varies from the description in the book, or if you learn of a program that you feel should be included in the book, please let us know.

The Common Sense of Weight Loss

In talking to people who have successfully lost weight and been able to maintain a healthy weight, I have heard an astonishing variety of approaches:

One woman lost weight on one program in this book, but couldn't maintain the loss until switching to a different program (one with which she initially had failed to lose weight).

A man chose the most expensive program he could find simply because he knew that having paid thousands of dollars to lose weight would provide him with the steadfast resolve he knew he needed. It worked!

A woman lost the first 15 pounds in the privacy of her own home with one of the liquid supplement programs before feeling good enough about herself to even show up at a public weight loss program. Then, slowly she lost the rest of the weight she wanted.

Another woman who gained weight on five different diets because her response to feeling deprived was to cheat and eat, gradually lost all the weight she had been trying so hard to lose simply by giving up diets altogether and resolving to eat in a healthy manner and not to deprive herself.

As these stories indicate, losing weight and keeping it off is a very personal matter. What works for one person will not work for another. Just as our body shapes and sizes, metabolisms, temperaments, and lifestyles differ, so what we need out of a weight loss program will be different for each of us. For some, good nutritional information and determination will be enough. For others a highly structured program is essential. Group meetings and support play a vital role in maintaining resolve for many, while others are so uncomfortable or embarrassed by group sessions that it can undermine their desire to continue. The trick is to figure out what approach or combinations of approaches works for you.

Right now there are quite a number of choices out there and that can be very confusing. This is particularly true when advertisements say very little about a particular approach and rely instead on testimonials. Most programs can provide valuable help but without details, it is not always clear which approach would be most beneficial for you.

The vast amount of dollars at stake in the weight loss industry has provided one very positive benefit for consumers: Competition among the various plans is very aggressive both in pricing and in attempts to continually upgrade programs in order to achieve the best results. Since most weight loss programs know that the best advertisements for their program are successful graduates, they have incentive for achieving good results.

In the infancy of these programs, that translated into "before" and "after" photos and simple, straightforward testimonials of recent graduates. However, the consuming public was quick to understand that all too often the slim, smiling testifiers regained the lost pounds after the ad was printed. So most programs were quick to respond with increased emphasis on what is now seen as the most important part of weight loss–keeping the pounds off after the diet ends.

Yet for all the differing programs and all the assurances of quick and lasting weight loss, it remains true that each of us gained our extra pounds on our own and we must each find our own best and most appropriate method for returning to a healthy weight. This will undoubtedly be accomplished when you have a clear idea of what you need and what you should avoid in order to achieve success.

So, when comparing the different programs and approaches to weight loss in DIET RIGHT, you should identify the range of personal issues that you need to address in order to increase your chances of successful weight loss and long term maintenance of a healthy weight. Here's a list of questions designed to help you identify the criteria necessary to make an informed decision:

Personal Weight Loss Criteria

1. Am I ready to take responsibility for my own weight loss problem?
2. Can I do it on my own or do I need a highly structured program to succeed?
3. Am I willing to pay to lose weight? If so, how much?
4. Do I need help in altering my eating habits?
5. Could I benefit from group discussions?
6. Do I need a built-in support system?
7. Can I lose weight if I have to do the shopping and control my own portions or would I do better with pre-packaged, calorie restricted foods?
8. Would it be easier for me to lose weight by largely avoiding real food altogether and using a liquid supplement?
9. Would I do better losing weight quickly even if it took more determination, and then trying to adjust to a lifestyle that would allow me to maintain that level?
10. Would I be better off losing weight gradually and working slowly toward a solid maintenance diet?
11. Do I need assistance in beginning and sticking to an exercise program?
12. Does my weight problem have a psychological basis, and if so how best can I deal with it?

13. Do I have a track record of failure in earlier attempts to lose weight?
14. If so, what were the specific problems I encountered? What was difficult for me?
15. Do I fully understand the behavioral and nutritional issues important to maintaining a healthy weight?
16. Are there any potential health problems that should influence how I lose weight?

Once you have the answers to these questions, you should read about each program with your personal answers in mind, searching for the one that is best suited to what you need.

Keep in mind, however, that the physician-based programs are not necessarily better than the others. Often people think that the average physician receives a great deal of training in nutrition. However, while a program's medical director may be a recognized expert in the field, the physicians administering the program may be no more knowledgeable about nutritional issues than the average person.

Also be aware that perhaps the greatest overall weakness within the entire weight loss industry is the lack of good, sound, regular exercise programs incorporated into their systems. In general, the importance of exercise is difficult to overstate. (For a more complete discussion of the reasons why, see the chapter on Dieting Basics.) While most of the programs do encourage exercise, and some go as far as providing videos or attempting to structure a program for you, virtually none actually put you through the paces by having you show up on a regular basis for exercise classes or training sessions.

Some programs even go as far as to suggest that while exercise is good, it isn't a "necessary" component to weight loss. Whether this is because an structured exercise program would be very time intensive and therefore increase the cost of the program, or simply because the industry fears that most people want to lose weight but are unwilling to exercise, is difficult to say. Hopefully, as competition within the industry heats up further and as reliable, independent figures become available as to the long term success rate of differing programs, we will see a more comprehensive structured introduction of exercise into weight loss programs. In the meantime, be aware that this is a dieting component that you will have to provide pretty much on your own.

Dieting Basics

What is a healthy weight? The Metropolitan Life Insurance Company has an answer that over the years has become the de facto guideline for "Ideal Body Weight." (Insurance companies are apparently queasy about people weighing in without clothing; you should note, therefore, that for the purpose of the following charts, weights and heights are calculated fully clothed. The Metropolitan Life chart assumes five pounds of clothing on a man wearing shoes with one-inch heels, and approximately three pounds of clothing for women wearing two-inch heels. Therefore, if you weigh yourself barefoot and in your birthday suit, men should add an inch to their height and subtract five pounds from the "ideal weights" while women should add two inches to their height and subtract three pounds to fit chart requirements.)

Metropolitan Life Insurance Company Height and Weight Tables

	Height	Small Frame	Med. Frame	Large Frame
Men	5'2"	128-134	131-141	138-150
	5'3"	130-136	133-143	140-153
	5'4"	132-138	135-145	142-156
	5'5"	134-140	137-148	144-160
	5'6"	136-142	139-151	146-164
	5'7"	138-145	142-154	149-168
	5'8"	140-148	145-157	152-172
	5'9"	142-151	148-160	155-176
	5'10"	144-154	151-163	158-180
	5'11"	146-157	154-166	161-184
	6'	149-160	157-170	164-188
	6'1"	152-164	160-174	168-192
	6'2"	155-168	164-178	172-197
	6'3"	158-172	167-182	176-202
	6'4"	162-176	171-187	181-207

	Height	Small Frame	Med. Frame	Large Frame
Women	4'10"	102-111	109-121	118-131
	4'11"	103-113	111-123	120-134
	5'	104-115	113-126	122-137
	5'1"	106-118	115-129	125-140
	5'2"	108-121	118-132	128-143
	5'3"	111-124	121-135	131-147
	5'4"	114-127	124-138	134-151
	5'5"	117-130	127-141	137-155
	5'6"	120-133	130-144	140-159
	5'7"	123-136	133-147	143-163
	5'8"	126-139	136-150	146-167
	5'9"	129-142	139-153	149-170
	5'10"	132-145	142-156	152-173
	5'11"	135-148	145-159	155-176
	6'	138-151	148-162	158-179

Now this may be a standard guideline but it's not the Bible. We are all blessed or cursed with a particular genetic inheritance and what may make sense for the Met Life models might look ridiculous on you, or worse, be impossible to maintain. Indeed, there is a growing concern that as a society we have tended to place too much emphasis on everyone meeting some arbitrary standard of slimness.

Perhaps that prompted the Society of Actuaries and Association of Life Insurance Medical Directors of America to develop their own chart. In 1979, they did a mortality study of four million healthy adults and came up with a range of weights at which you could expect to live a long and healthy life. Like the folks at Met Life they preferred weighing people with clothes on, so for the following chart naked men should add one inch to their height and subtract five pounds. Since fashions have changed and high heels were less in evidence during this study, women should add only one inch to compensate for the absence of shoes and subtract three pounds to arrive at their unclothed weight.

	Height	Small Frame	Med. Frame	Large Frame
Men	5'2"	128-134	131-141	138-150
	5'3"	130-136	133-143	140-153
	5'4"	132-138	135-145	142-156
	5'5"	134-140	137-148	144-160
	5'6"	136-142	139-151	146-164
	5'7"	138'145	142-154	149-168
	5'8"	140-148	145-157	152-172
	5'9"	142-151	148-160	155-176
	5'10"	144-154	151-163	158-180
	5'11"	146-157	154-166	161-184
	6'	149-160	157-170	164-188
	6'1"	152-164	160-174	168-192
	6'2"	155-168	164-178	172-197
	6'3"	158-172	167-182	176-202
	6'4"	162-176	171-187	181-207
	Height	**Small Frame**	**Med. Frame**	**Large Frame**
Women	4'10"	102-111	109-121	118-131
	4'11"	103-113	111-123	120-134
	5'	104-115	113-126	122-137
	5'1"	106-118	115-129	125-140
	5'2"	108-121	118-132	128-143
	5'3"	111-124	121-135	131-147
	5'4"	114-127	124-138	134-151
	5'5"	117-130	127-141	137-155
	5'6"	120-133	130-144	140-159
	5'7"	123-136	133-147	143-163
	5'8"	126-139	136-150	146-167
	5'9"	129-142	139-153	149-170
	5'10"	132-145	142-156	152-173
	5'11"	135-148	145-159	155-176
	6'	138-151	148-162	158-179

Another way to estimate your Ideal Body Weight utilized by dietitians is the quick and easy method. For women, start with 100 pounds for the first five feet of height, and then add five pounds for every additional inch of height. For men start with 106 pounds for the first five feet of height and then add six pounds for every additional inch of height. In both cases, the resulting weight will be your ideal body weight plus or minus ten percent.

Changing ideas about what is an Ideal Body Weight, however, cannot hide the fact that seriously overweight individuals are placing themselves at serious health risk for a wide assortment of problems. Just how much weight is too much in terms of health risk is difficult to assess, but those who medically qualify as obese have definitely crossed that line. The medical definition of obese is 20 percent more than Ideal Body Weight; if a person is 100 pounds over Ideal Body Weight, he or she is considered morbidly obese and more than likely already is experiencing serious health-related problems.

In determining your own appropriate weight, you should take the Ideal Body Weight charts into consideration, and understand that crossing the line into obesity carries considerable health risks. However, rather than just blindly trying to fit into an "Ideal Body Weight" model, you should find a weight at which you feel comfortable and that can be maintained with relative ease, one that can allows you to pursue an active lifestyle and feel good about yourself.

The Truth about Weight Loss

Despite the hundreds of diets, gadgets, pills, and magic elixirs sold over the years to help people lose weight, the body continues to respond to its own basic truth: If you consume more calories than you burn off you gain weight; if you eat fewer calories than you burn off you lose weight; if you consume the same amount of calories as you burn off you maintain your current weight.

Like the practitioners of alchemy in the Middle Ages, modern day enthusiasts have sought numerous ways around the laws of nature, but to no avail. Our bodies are like wonderfully complex and highly tuned machines that use food as fuel. In the case of food, the "octane ratings" of different food can be found in readily available calorie tables. Once we have eaten and begun to digest the calories consumed, our bodies only know two ways to deal with the new calories we have taken in. They can use them to keep us going or store them as fat.

That is why to lose weight there are only three things you can do that will be effective: Consume fewer calories, burn off more calories through exercise while keeping your caloric intake at the same level, or exercise and eat fewer calories.

How many calories are required in order to keep someone at a healthy weight will vary with each individual. Because we are all distinct, our bodies all operate slightly differently. Also, how active we are will greatly affect the number of calories we need to maintain our current weight. Exercise burns calories. For example, a man aged 35 who weighs 150 pounds and is moderately active might burn between 2400 and 2600 calories per day, while a women of the same age, weight and activity level would burn between 1900 and 2200 calories In addition, the heavier you are the more calories you will use in a day, and the older you get the fewer calories you will use.

What no doubt comes to mind immediately is that once you lose weight and achieve the weight level you feel comfortable with, the amount of calories you can consume to stay at that level, assuming your activity level remain the same, is less that what you currently consume. Therein is the primary explanation for the yo-yo syndrome–the frustrating cycle of losing weight and then putting it right back on again.

To slightly oversimplify, one pound of fat is the

equivalent of 3500 calories. Therefore, if, at your pre-diet weight level you were burning 2,800 calories per day without losing or gaining weight and now at your new weight level you are burning only 2,300 calories per day (remember it takes more energy, i.e., more calories, to keep a heavier body functioning), then in one week you will have burned 3500 fewer calories that you used to (7 x 500). That's why, if after you reached your new desired weight, you'll simply return to eating the same foods in the same amounts as before, you end up gaining back one pound each week until you return to your pre-diet weight.

Metabolism and Weight Loss

Number of calories is not the whole issue. Metabolism also plays a vital role in both losing and gaining weight. In laypersons' terms, metabolism is simply the level at which our bodies uses energy and burns calories. In recent years, metabolism has been much discussed, with claims and confusion predominating over facts. Indeed, several new diets have recently emerged that are based on the premise that your metabolism can be fooled into burning more calories than it otherwise would. Unfortunately your metabolism isn't that stupid, and any diet that claims to be able to fool your metabolism is really just trying to fool you.

To be perfectly fair, the confusion was not simply the result of overaggressive advertising of "new and exciting" ways to lose weight. Like much of our knowledge in the area of nutrition and weigh loss, the picture is only now beginning to become clear.

Indeed until very recently, even among the scientific community it was believed that prolonged periods on Very Low Calorie Diets or even the cumulative experience of undertaking too many diets would permanently reset your metabolism at lower levels. This is a frightening thought for anyone trying to lose weight, since it raises the horrible image of eating fewer calories, thereby forever lowering your metabolism. You burn fewer calories so the calories in/calories out formula never catches up until you feel like you are starving to death and not losing a pound.

What made this fear all the more worrisome was that this theory was based on a certain amount of common sense and experience. Whenever people begin a diet, their bodies respond to the lowered intake of calories by lowering the rate at which they burn calories. This is not an unreasonable response since as far as our bodies' automatic monitoring system can tell, we appear to be short of food. Our bodies are simply working in the interest of our long-term survival by slowing our metabolism to preserve what calories it can.

Therefore, the more restrictive the diet, the greater the drop in metabolism. In tests carried on with people on very low calorie diets, metabolism rates dropped dramatically. This is one of the reasons that it often feels like the amount of food you are restricted to on a diet should be generating much more dramatic weight loss that it actually does.

According to the then-prevalent theory, once you arrive at your desired weight, your metabolism remains permanently artificially lowered and you must remain on a diet of dramatically fewer calories in order to keep from regaining not only the weight you lost, but even more.

Fortunately, although the final word is not yet in, the body does not appear to be such a cruel master. Recent studies indicate that while any dieting will result in an immediate lowering of your metabolism, it will bounce back to a level appropriate for your new, stabilized weight. That level will, of course, be lower than your pre-diet level since you now weigh less and therefore it takes less energy to get your body through the day, but your metabolism will return to a level consistent with your new weight. The chart below provides a rough example of the effect of dieting and weight loss on a typical dieter's metabolism.

Mildly active 150 pound woman

Amount consumed	
per day:	+2200 calories
resting metabolism:	-1300 calories
light activity:	- 900 calories

0 pounds gained or lost

After beginning a moderate calorie diet :	
amount consumed:	+1100 calories:
resting metabolism	
decreases to around:	-900 calories
light activity:	-900 calories

-700 calories per day

Even though the dieter in the example above has cut back the calories she consumes by 1000 calories, because her metabolism slowed down when she began to diet her daily calorie "deficit" is only 700 calories.

So far, all the studies indicating that your metabolic rate will rebound after your diet is completed, have involved participants who have been exercising regularly, so perhaps the message here is to make sure regular exercise is an element of your daily life. Indeed the relationship between metabolism and exercise is very important, partly because of the way the body's metabolism works to get the energy to keep functioning.

Why Exercise is Important

Weight loss diets are all structured so that you consume fewer calories than you use, and while this process alone will result in weight loss, the kind of weight being lost is significant. This is because, faced with fewer calories coming in as food, your body turns first to stored carbohydrates (glycogen) for energy, and as a second choice burns off the protein that makes up our lean muscle mass. It is only as a third choice that fat is metabolized. On the other hand, good aerobic exercise gets the oxygen into the body's cells, which has the effect of directly metabolizing stored fat.

In short, a diet without exercise is liable to result in weight loss but with much of the loss coming from lean muscle mass rather than body fat. This then poses an additional problem since we end up with a smaller percentage of our bodies composed of lean muscle mass and therefore with a lower metabolic level than would be true if we had maintained our previous percentage of lean muscle mass. That's because one other quirk of metabolism is that the greater the percentage of our bodies that is muscle mass, the higher our metabolism. This poses an additional difficulty for women–since men normally have a greater muscle mass than women, a man weighing 140 pounds will tend to burn more calories than a women of the same weight doing the same activity. Thus women have to exercise more to burn the same amount of calories as men, although as they exercise and get more muscle mass, the gap closes.

What all of this means is that a diet combined with a good aerobic exercise regime will tend to burn off more pounds from stored fat than lean muscle mass, thereby increasing the percentage of lean muscle mass in our bodies which in turn will help to increase our metabolic rate so we burn calories more efficiently.

In fact, the good news relative to metabolism is that exercise increases the rate at which you burn calories--not only on a short-term basis but overall. A recent study of college wrestlers demonstrated some promising results. The wrestlers had gone through at least three different annual cycles of losing weight in order to qualify for specified weight divisions, followed by an extended period of training during the season, followed by weight gain after the season. They were compared to men of approximately the same age and size that were used as a control group.

The study found that the wrestlers started with a significantly higher resting metabolic rate (i.e., the "couch potato" rate when they were at rest and not involved in any activity) than the control group. Then during weight loss, their resting metabolism rate decreased, but not significantly lower than that of the control group. Once the season was over and they had regained their weight their resting metabolic levels returned to the previous level–above that of the control group.

This study not only demonstrated that the lower metabolism rates common to dieting will rebound once the diet is over, but also showed the long-term beneficial effect of exercise in raising metabolic levels. Thus, dieters who engage in regular invigorating exercise will speed weight loss without any extra calorie deprivation simply by elevating their metabolic rates. This is particularly true in cases where a dieter is making the transition from a very sedentary lifestyle to one of gradually increased activity.

However, any activity will burn calories, and the more strenuous the activity the more calories will be burned. For example, an hour's worth of leisurely bike riding or an hour of dragging your clubs around a golf course will burn off around 300 calories (the equivalent of a McDonalds' cheeseburger, a couple beers or a cream puff). The chart below lists a number of common activities and a rough estimate of the number of calories consumed per hour of activity.

Calories Used Per Minute

Climbing stairs	8-10
Cycling (casually)	4-5
Cycling (vigorously)	11
Dancing	4-7
Football	10
Golf	5
Jogging	11
Jumping Rope	15-20
Rowing	12-19
Running	18-20
Skiing	15
Sweeping	4
Swimming	7-11
Tennis	7-10
Walking	3-5

The bottom line is that regular exercise is probably the single most effective way to lose weight and if that exercise is aerobic, you get the extra benefit of a direct health dividend to your cardiovascular system. Aerobic exercise is any exercise that get your heart pumping in the range of 70% to 85% of your maximum heart rate. To receive the benefit from such exercise, you should do aerobic exercises for a minimum of 20 minutes at a time, for a minimum of three times a week.

A simple way to determine what is the proper heart rate for your aerobic exercise is to subtract your age from 220 to get your maximum heart rate in beats per minute. Then multiply that figure by .70 and .85 to get your aerobic range. For example, a 20 year old's maximum heart rate will be 200 beats per minute (220 minus 20). Multiply that by .70 and .85 and you get an aerobic range of between 140 and 170 beats per minute. So when a 20-year-old does aerobic exercise, his or her heart rate should be between 140 and 170 beats per minute.

Expand Your Food Horizons

To risk overstretching the metaphor, our bodies require considerably more than pure calories in order to operate at peak effectiveness; we also require all the additives supplied by key nutrients such as vitamins and minerals. Therefore, when we fuel up we must do so with a eye toward getting all the nutrients we need. The official list of what the best scientific research thinks we need is contained in the U.S. Recommended Daily Allowances, frequently shown as U.S. RDA or just RDA:

Recommended Dietary Allowances (RDA)

	Male age 23-50 154 lbs., 5'10"	Female age 23-50 120 lbs., 5'4"
Protein	56 grms	44 grms
Vitamin A	1000 µg RE	800 µg RE
Vitamin D	5 µg	5 µg
Vitamin E	10 mg	8 mg
VitaminC	60 mg	60 mg
Thiamin	1.4 mg	1.0 mg
Roboflavin	1.6 mg	1.2 mg
Niacin	18 mgNE	13 mg NE
Vitamin B-6	2.2 mg	2.0 mg
Folacin	400 µg	400 µg
Calcium	3.0 µg	3.0 µg
Phosphorus	800 mg	800 mg
Magnesium	350 mg	300 mg
Iron	10 mg	18 mg
Zinc	15 mg	15 mg
Iodine	150 µg	150 µg

You can spend hours per day comparing charts containing the source and amounts of nutrients in foods with the RDA chart above, but it is much simpler to intelligently choose the food you eat. If you do so, and if you follow some fairly simple guidelines, you will automatically satisfy your nutritional requirements, eat a healthier diet, and almost certainly consumer fewer calories than you currently do.

The first consideration is to try to fit your diet into the macro-nutritional breakdown recommended by the U.S. Department of Health: Total calories should equal 12 percent protein, 30 percent fat and 58 percent carbohydrate (with a heavy emphasis on complex carbohydrates). Since most Americans currently consume around 42 percent of their calories in fat and only 46 percent in carbohydrates (and this mostly in the simple sugar category rather than the complex grains category), there is much room for improvement.

Secondly, you should attempt to eat a wide variety of foods in the proportions shown below:

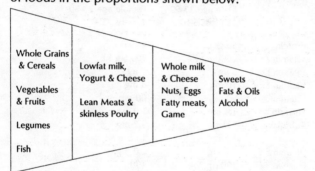

Whole Grains & Cereals	Lowfat milk, Yogurt & Cheese	Whole milk & Cheese Nuts, Eggs	Sweets Fats & Oils
Vegetables & Fruits	Lean Meats & skinless Poultry	Fatty meats, Game	Alcohol
Legumes			
Fish			

You should choose liberally from foods to the left in the above diagram and as the triangle narrows, increasingly cut back the amounts of these foods. If you can balance out your diet in this fashion, you should have no trouble assuring yourself of a sound and balanced diet.

You Are What You Feel

Lastly, but far from least, you should consider not only the calorie content, but the emotional significance of food. Food is a powerful actor in our emotional lives. It not only provides us with the means of physical survival, but it is seductive and pleasurable. It should not be surprising, therefore, that an increasing number of weight loss specialists have targeted the emotional issues surrounding food as one of the prime culprits in overweight and particularly obese individuals.

When food becomes a substitute for love or attention, a coping mechanism for stress and discomfort, or a refuge for escape, the results are almost always hard on the body and even more difficult to unwind and escape from. Returning to and maintaining a healthy weight may well be predicated upon facing up to personal psychological problems. Many of the programs in this book attempt to deal with the psychological issues surrounding overeating. Additionally, there are many good books on the subject–see page 24 for a list of some of them.

Four Approaches to Losing Weight

Slow and Easy: Perhaps the most common theory held by dietitians and other specialists in the field is that weight should be lost in the reverse manner from which it was gained: slowly and through sound eating habits. According to the American Dietetic Association, the best pound per week loss rate is approximately one-half to two-thirds pound.

This can be accomplished simply by doing two things–eating properly and getting off your duff to begin even a moderate exercise regime. The premise (and unfortunately a usually correct one) is that virtually everyone who is overweight is guilty of two sins: 1. eating too much of the wrong foods and too little of the right foods; and 2. living an overly sedentary lifestyle. Simply changing eating habits to a more healthy diet and beginning to exercise will result in a moderate calorie deficiency that will, over time, bring your weight back to a stable and healthy level.

The advantage of this approach is that the entire

time you are losing weight you are also learning how to keep your weight at a healthy level. As just about anyone who has dieted will tell you, losing weight is not difficult at all compared with maintaining the weight loss.

The down side to the slow and easy method is that it can take six to nine months to lose 20 pounds and it requires both a good understanding of what diet changes need to be made as well as the ability to implement those changes without major backsliding.

Moderate Dieting: For many, the slow and easy method is both too slow and not so easy since it requires a lot of self-motivation, self-discipline, and commitment on a daily basis. For those people a more structured dieting program that aims to shed one to two pounds per week and includes some outside assistance and support may be a good idea.

The advantage of this approach is that you can get all the assistance, information, and support you need, you will see results faster which will hopefully translate into greater resolve, and you will not have to rely completely on yourself to keep to the straight and narrow or return to the straight and narrow after a side trip to the candy store. The disadvantage is that it may make your transition from weight loss to weight maintenance slightly more difficult since the natural tendency after weeks or months of dieting is to want to "return to normal" eating patterns.

Hide the Food Dieting: Slow or moderate methods may not be the best approach for obese or seriously obese individuals. That is because at some point, the quantity of extra pounds you are carrying around poses a greater health risk in and of itself than the potential problems with very rapid weight loss. If you are in this situation you should read the chapter on Very Low Calorie Diets carefully.

The advantage of Very Low Calorie Diets (they are almost always diets that totally replace food with fortified formula drinks and soups) is that you lose weight at a very rapid pace. For someone with 50 to 100 pounds to lose this can be critical since otherwise it could literally take years of near perfect dieting to return to a healthy weight.

Another possible advantage is that by going completely without food, you have a clean break from what were clearly very poor food habits. The disadvantage is that there can be health risks associated with such a rapid weight loss, and it may be very difficult to develop the kinds of new food habits that will be necessary to keep the weight from returning without actually practicing them for extended periods of time.

When Diets Don't Work: For some people, none of the above methods is likely to result in anything but frustration and a deteriorating self-image. For too many people food and their emotional lives have become so tangled together that any attempts to reduce by dieting will only set in motion a vicious cycle of failure. The very idea of dieting can trigger increased feelings of deprivation, stress, depression, or anger–the very feelings that all too often drive people to eat in the first place. This approach advocates giving up the concept of dieting and discover what is behind cravings for food.

There are a number of books that deal with various aspects of this issue including *Making Peace with Food* by Susan Kano, *Overcoming Overeating* by Jane Hirshmann & Carol Munter, *Feeding the Hungry Heart* and *When Food is Love* by Geneen Roth, *It's Not What You're Eating, It's What's Eating You* by Janet Greeson, *Listen to the Hunger: Why we Overeat* by Elisabeth L, and *Fat is a Feminist Issue* by Susie Orbach.

Very Low Calorie Diets

Over the past ten years, one of the most controversial subjects in the dieting world has been the safety and advisability of what has come to be called Very Low Calorie Diets (VLCDs) that are usually available in liquid supplement form. In part, the controversy surrounding these diets stems from the unfortunate, premature commercial availability of a number of diets in the late 1970s that led to a significant number of reported deaths at least partially attributed to the diets themselves.

Given the history of weight loss scams in this country, the tragic result of a rush to profit from the newest "miracle" diets was probably as predictable as it was unfortunate. The tragedy was only enhanced by the fact that the nutritional breakthrough inherent in the development of the Very Low Calorie Diets is of potentially major significance, particularly for those people suffering from serious obesity.

For decades, because of the increasing evidence of the cumulative health risks associated with seriously obese individuals, medical researchers have sought an effective way to promote rapid weight loss. They soon discovered a "fact" that intuitively the world has known all along: Starvation is a very effective way to lose weight. The first major clinical trial of such an idea was conducted in 1959 by W.L. Bloom with nine patients who fasted for one week and lost 18.5 pounds "with ease." That encouraged a wave of new clinical trials in 1960 that proved equally effective.

Fortunately for the public, fasting never made it big in the marketplace. By 1970 a number of deaths related to fasting were reported, and it was discovered that much of the weight lost on a fast came from lean body mass rather than fat since that was the simplest way for the body to find usable calories in the absence of food. Even worse, once the fast ended, the weight had a tendency to reappear, this time as more fat, almost as rapidly as it had fallen away.

It was at this juncture that attention turned to the development of a Very Low Calorie Diet. The theory was that since on average individuals burn between 1700 and 2100 calories per day, a diet of less that 800 calories would promote rapid weight loss but would continue to supply enough protein to preserve lean body mass. Attempts were made in 1966 to develop liquid protein supplements, but the lack of complete nutritional information led to further problems.

The issue came to a head in the late 1970s. Between 1976 and 1978, the most widely known and available liquid protein diet, The Last Chance Diet, was used to some degree by over 100,000 people. By 1978, the Food and Drug Administration and the Centers for Disease Control had received reports of over 60 deaths related to liquid protein diets, mostly The Last Chance Diet.

In following up on the reported deaths, researchers found that the primary cause of death was heart failure, that the majority of victims had pre-existing illnesses, and that they had existed only on the liquid protein diet for at least four months. While this was disturbing news, the most distressing finding was that 17 of the deaths had occurred to relatively young people with no pre-existing illnesses.

Medical researchers have done an extensive postmortem on those early diets and there is a general consensus that the diets responsible for those deaths suffered a number of serious nutritional deficiencies, including the use of a low quality protein, the absence of elements necessary to balance out the nitrogen levels in the body, and a deficiency in numerous other elements and minerals necessary for the healthy functioning of the human body.

Since the national scare sparked by the Last Chance Diet, the medical community has gotten a handle on the crucial nutritional components of Very Low Calorie Diets. The VLCDs of today are very different from their predecessors. They consist of complete proteins of very high biological value with recommended dosages of between 50 and 100 grams of protein per day. Most consist of a powdered preparation from egg, milk, or soy base that can be mixed with water or other liquids to make drinks or soups. Supplemented with vitamins, minerals, and electrolytes to bring them up to 100 percent of U.S. Recommended Daily Allowances, they also contain carbohydrates and flavoring to make them more palatable. Taken three to five times daily, the formulas usually supply between 400 and 800 calories per day.

There is a general consensus that the new generation of VLCDs are safe when administered under the proper circumstances. However, there is still some disagreement about what those circumstances are. The highly respected American Dietetic Association (ADA) suggests that, because of the potential health risks associated with VLCDs, the appropriate candidates for VLCDs should be carefully screened by a health care team consisting of a physician knowledgeable about weight loss issues, a registered dietitian, and a behavioral therapist.

The ADA also believes that the degree of obesity is an important safety factor. They point to studies that demonstrate both a greater degree of heart problems and a higher rate of body protein loss associated with lighter individuals on VLCDs. Thus, the thinner you are, the more problems such a diet could cause. On the other hand, as obesity increases, the health risks of obesity itself become more dominant; that is, it may be more dangerous to remain severely overweight than to use a VLCD. Therefore the ADA recommends that VLCDs only be used with dieters who are at least 30 percent overweight.

The ADA also recommends without exception that VLCDs not be used for infants, children, adolescents, pregnant or breastfeeding mothers, patients who have had cardiac failure or myocardial infarction within six months, or patients with active cancer, hepatic disease, renal failure, or severe psychological disturbances.

If a VLCD is used, the ADA recommends that dieters carefully evaluate the administering program to assure there is adequate physician monitoring, nutrition counseling, a behavioral component, and an exercise program.

Not everyone agrees with the ADA's position. Some medical researchers and certainly many of the medical directors of programs offering VLCDs claim that the latest formulas have been demonstrated to be very safe under a much broader use than that recommended by the ADA. They argue that the benefits and advantages of VLCDs should not be denied to healthy individuals who are not necessarily 30 percent overweight. Almost everyone, however, agrees that anyone using a VLCD should be carefully monitored by a physician who is familiar with the possible side effects (such as dehydration, electrolyte imbalance, headaches, muscle cramps, minor hair loss, gastrointestinal distress, and intolerance to cold) as well as the potentially more serious problems associated with such diets.

Another issue that has surrounded the debate on VLCDs is the relative advantages and disadvantages of dieting without eating. Some proponents of the VLCD formulas claim that it is easier for obese individuals to completely forego solid food than it is to limit the kind and quantity they can eat. According to this theory, rather than tempt yourself at every meal, it is simpler to just swear off food altogether until your weight is down to an appropriate level. Another argument is that VLCDs are a way to make a dramatic break with what were obviously bad eating habits in the hope that a clean start will follow when the dieter returns to grocery store food.

Opponents believe that the kind of behavioral changes that are necessary in order to keep from regaining all the weight that was lost cannot be accomplished very easily without the kind of long-term practice that a more conventional diet requires. According to this theory, no amount of lectures and handouts will

31

break the old ingrained habits; it has to be practiced.

In the final analysis, the decision must be made by the consumer, since at the present time, there are no licensing boards preventing the marketplace from offering VLCDs to anyone interested, and what will work for one person may not work for another. Virtually all of the currently operating VLCD weight loss programs attempt to determine if there are any possible health conditions that might increase the risks associated with dieting, and most advise their customers to seek the advice of their physician, particularly before participating in a VLCD. Additionally, most programs have introduced transition periods and maintenance programs that are designed to retrain dieters to proper eating habits.

The best approach is to be fully informed. Be sure to consult your personal physician, seek advice from professionals if you need it, and be realistic about what will and will not work for you.

Moderate Calorie/Grocery Store Food Programs

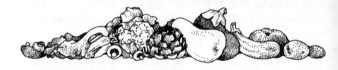

The Diet Center

The Diet Center grew out of the personal experience of its founder, Sybil Ferguson. In 1970, after years of failed attempts to lose weight, Sybil Ferguson found herself 58 pounds overweight, suffering from malnutrition, and forced to put off necessary surgery because her overweight condition made it too dangerous.

Determined to finally lose the weight and keep it off, she educated herself and, with the help of her doctor, developed her own diet plan which proved effective. After slimming down to a healthy weight, she began to share her ideas with friends in Rexburg, ID. Local physicians heard of her success and began referring overweight patients to her. Thus began what is today one of the largest weight loss programs in the world; over 2300 Diet Centers are spread across the United States, Canada, Australia, and England.

HOW IT WORKS: The Diet Center operates what it calls a five-phase program: Conditioning, Reducing, Sta.b.lite., Maintenance, and Image One. Upon registering, you complete a health review questionnaire. If health issues arise in the answers, The Diet Center either contacts your doctor, or has you talk to your doctor. For those who are 40 percent or more overweight, need to lose 50 pounds or more, or have any pre-existing health problems, a complete physical examination and doctor's approval is required before beginning.

The Conditioning Phase lasts two days, and is meant to prepare you both mentally and physically for the regime to follow. During this phase you are restricted to a moderate calorie diet of the basic food groups that will be used throughout the reducing phase. You also begin taking Diet Center Supplement tablets, fortified food products with B complex vitamins in a base of soy protein meant to assist in alleviating hunger.

During the Reducing Phase, you stick to the Diet Center diet of around 1000 calories for women and 1250 calories for men and meet daily with a Diet Center Counselor. The Counselor provides personal support and encouragement throughout your progress, and serves as your personal advisor with helpful information, tips, and nutritional assistance.

You also begin attending weekly meetings of the Phase Five Image One Series, where issues such as nutritional education, behavior modification, self-direction, stress management and exercise are discussed. The goal of the Image One Series is to provide the information necessary to make intelligent, informed decisions relative to long-term weight control. The Reducing Phase continues until you reach your goal weight.

Then you shift to the Sta.b.lite Phase during which sessions with your counselor continue three time per week. During this period, which typically lasts nine weeks, caloric intake is gradually increased to around 1400 calories for women and 1700 for men. The purpose is to find the appropriate level of calories and balance of nutritional elements to allow you to maintain your weight loss without hunger.

During the Maintenance Phase, your caloric intake is increased to levels designed to maintain healthy weight, and you are encouraged to continue to attend weekly Image One meetings for a full year. The maintenance phase can be extended as long as you feel necessary, with a once-a-week meeting with your Counselor.

THE DIET: The underlying principle of The Diet Center is that a stable blood sugar level is crucial to the success of any diet. According to the Diet Center, low blood sugar triggers a hungry response, which is all too often met with the ingestion of some form of refined sugar. While the immediate response is a rapid rise in blood sugar, it also drops quickly, leaving you hungry again. In addition a rapid rise in blood sugar can cause excess production of insulin which encourages the body to store the sugar as fat. Unfortunately, there is little in the way of reliable research to substantiate this theory.

The Diet Center program is designed to avoid a blood sugar roller coaster by eliminating refined sugar completely and providing dieters with a carefully scheduled diet of complex carbohydrates which, it says, allows blood sugar levels to rise and fall much more gradually.

The Diet itself begins with the two-day Conditioning Phase in which you are allowed daily unlimited servings of lean protein and vegetables, two servings of grains, five to seven servings of fruit and two teaspoons of fat daily. You also take eight tablets per day of the B complex supplement.

During the Reducing Phase, you eat seven to nine ounces of lean protein, two large servings of vegetables, two large servings of fruit, two servings of grains, two teaspoons of fat and eight tablets of the Diet Center B-Complex Supplement daily. This diet is maintained until you reach your goal weight.

Then, during the Stabilization phase you gradually increase you calorie intake first by increasing your protein levels to 12 to 14 ounces per day and your vegetables to two to four large servings per day plus a cup of some dairy product. Eventually you reach a level adequate to maintain your weight.

The nutritional breakdown of the Diet Center diet is 27 percent protein, 23 percent fat, and 50 percent carbohydrate for the reducing diet, and 19-22 percent protein, 26-28 percent fat and 52-53 percent carbohydrates at the maintenance phase.

SUPPLEMENTAL PRODUCTS: The Diet Center does not require you to purchase packaged foods; however, it does offer a wide variety of convenience products. These include sweeteners, spices, sauces, salad dressings, drinks, breads, protein powder, and breath mints.

STAFF: For the most part, the staff is composed of people who have successfully completed the Diet Center program and have been trained by The Diet Center to help guide other overweight individuals to a successful conclusion. The Diet Center only selects staff members who have been overweight and been successful in their program, because it believes that personal experience is an invaluable aid to helping others lose weight.

COST: Approximately $40 per week during the Reducing Phase and gradually decreasing for the other phases. For example, to lose 30 pounds would cost around $750.

AVERAGE WEIGHT LOSS: Approximately two and a half to three pounds per week.

PERSONAL CONSIDERATIONS: The Diet Center is a program that teaches you how to lose weight and maintain that loss while continuing to shop at the grocery store. This may make it easier for you to make the transition to normal life than it would using programs that use either packaged foods or formulated products exclusively. It may, however, be difficult for some people to properly control serving portions and shopping behavior with this program. For those who feel the need to get out of the grocery store and the kitchen during the reducing phase, this may not be the best plan for you.

Because The Diet Center offers so many supplemental products, it can be used as a kind of grocery store/pre-packaged food program. That might make a difference for those who don't feel they have the time to properly prepare shopping lists and carefully select, cook, and measure out serving portions.

The Diet Center does offer daily counseling during the reducing phase of the program, and for those people who know that they are going to need lots of help and encouragement, this is one feature that could be very important. However, the counseling is done by trained graduates of the program rather than health care providers, registered dietitians, or psychologists, and depending on your needs, this could pose a problem.

LOCATION: Available nationwide. The location nearest you can be found by writing The Diet Center, 921 Penn Ave., 9th Floor, Pittsburgh PA 15222 or by calling (412) 338-8700.

The Diet Workshop

The Diet Workshop is the product of a woman who described herself as a "fat child, a fat teenager and a fat adult." In 1964, Lois Lindauer, the owner and inspiration for The Diet Workshop, went on an eight-month mission to gain control over her weight; she ended up 42 pounds thinner and determined to help others do the same. She conducted her first weight control classes to 18 participants in the apartment of a friend in Boston. By 1967 she had refined her approach, expanded her territory, and sold the first of more than 30 franchise offices of The Diet Workshop.

Today, The Diet Workshop serves around 25,000 members a week primarily in the northeastern and midwest states but with locations in Texas, Florida and Kentucky as well. Lindauer has also authored four books dealing with weight loss: *It's In to Be Thin* (1970); *The Fast and Easy Teenage Diet* (1973); *The Diet Workshop Success Diet* (1978); and *The Wild Weekend Diet* (1985).

HOW IT WORKS: The Diet Workshop offers four separate programs. You choose the one that's right for you. Each is based on what The Diet Workshop calls the "5 star Flexi-Diet," a system of food units you combine to make your own meals.

Flexi-Groups: This program involves private weekly weigh-ins and one-hour group meetings led by successful graduates of the program. Here members are given nutritional information and suggestions for behavioral changes, told about the importance of exercise, and supported in their efforts by inspirational weight loss success stories. (For those with a busy schedule The Diet Workshop is also offering Express Flex-Groups that meet for only 30 minutes per week.) Meetings are held at Diet Workshop locations or at other sites arranged by the local franchise.

Quick Loss Clinics: For an emphasis on fast weight loss, there is a more personal and intensive approach. This program includes a weekly weigh-in and a one-hour discussion in small groups of not more than 15 led by a staff moderator. The discussion groups stress behavior modification for weight control and focus on personal eating habits that can get in the way of maintaining a healthy weight. The diet used for this program is a variation of the 5 Star Flexi-Diet called Quick Loss 2000.

Workplace Program: The Workplace Program is designed for companies that want to offer a weight loss program on location either during the lunch hour or before or after working hours. It is based on the Workplace Wellness Diet. That again is a variation on the 5 Star Flexi-Diet but is structured in three phases and geared especially for working people. The program includes eight weekly meetings where nutritional information and behavior modification are discussed. Emphasis is also placed on issues surrounding diet and the working person such as stress management, how to eat in restaurants, and tips for brown bagging.

Person to Person: In this individualized program, you and a counselor design a diet to meet your personal needs and meet weekly to discuss any specific issues you may want to resolve in order to successfully attain and maintain a healthy weight.

THE DIET: The 5 Star Flexi-Diet is low in fat, sugar, and salt, and consists of three meals a day of proteins and carbohydrates. It is based on lists of interchangeable food "units" from which you choose. The food units are spelled out in materials provided by The Diet Workshop and serve the function of pre-determining calorie counts while retaining some flexibility as to what specifically is eaten. In this manner, the diet attempts to teach you to make intelligent choices from the outset.

The Diet Workshop provides fairly extensive lists of acceptable foods under its food unit system. The following list is just a sampling:

One Protein Unit equals 1 oz. of hard cheese, chicken, fish, shellfish, and turkey, and beef, pork, and lamb restricted to twice weekly;

One Grain Unit equals 1 oz. of bread or 1/2 cup of pasta, hot cereal, rice, and chinese noodles.

Fruit Units include specific amounts of most fruits including 1 medium apple, 1/2 banana, 1/2 grapefruit, a medium peach, and 1 cup of watermelon.

Dairy Units include 1 cup low-fat yogurt, 1 cup skim milk, and a packet for a diet milk shake.

Lo-Vegetables, which can be eaten without restriction, include asparagus, broccoli, cucumber, eggplant, lettuce, peppers, spinach, and zucchini.

Hi-Vegetables (1 Unit=1/2 cup): Baked beans, lentils, cooked onions, corn, potato, and tomato sauce.

The program starts with the Core Diet which averages around 1000 calories per day. This consists of:

Breakfast: 1 Protein Unit & 1 Grain Unit.

Lunch: 3 Protein Units, 1 Grain Unit, and any unlimited Lo-Vegetable.

Dinner: 4 Protein Units, 1 Hi-Vegetable Unit, unlimited Lo-Vegetables and 1 Grain Unit or 1 Fruit Unit or 1 Dairy Unit.

Added to this core diet are from one to ten additional units depending on your age, sex, and height.

In the second week, the Core Diet is supplemented with additional food units called the Core Booster Diet, to reach a daily caloric average of 1100. By week three the available choices are expanded and supplemented to attain a 1200 calorie per day program. At this time the program also allows what it calls Meal Exchange, which is a list of fast food items that can be substituted once for lunch and once for dinner each week. Included on that list are such things as a McDonald's cheeseburger, two slices of cheese pizza, a Dairy Queen hot dog, and a variety of frozen entrees.

The Diet Workshop recommends you supplement your nutritional needs while participating in the program with vitamins and minerals to round out your nutritional requirements and offers its own versions: eight Diet-Tabs (B-complex vitamin in soy protein) per day and a Vita/Mineral Pak.

SUPPLEMENTAL PRODUCTS: The Diet Workshop does not require participants to purchase its products; however, it does offer some items to complement its program. These include six pre-packaged dinners (Chili, Pasta Italiano, A La King, Fettuccine Roma, Sweet 'n Sour and Hearty Stew). It also sells a breakfast bar, three packaged soups, five low-calorie salad dressings, ten flavors of low-calorie candy, and a whole wheat and plum snack. The soy-based B-complex Diet-Tabs and the Vita/Mineral Paks recommended as part of the diet are also available.

The Diet Workshop's latest product is a 60-minute audio cassette packaged with an instructional hand-book on Fitness Walking.

STAFF: Like a number of other programs, the Diet Workshop uses trained graduates of the program. In addition to their original training, staff members meets monthly with program directors to go over new infor-mation.

COST: The Flexi-Group program costs $14 to register and $9 per meeting; a six week Quick Loss is under $70. Person to Person is $135 for a four-week program. The cost of the Workplace Program will depend on your employer. Some companies offer the program as a benefit; others ask for co-payment.

AVERAGE WEIGHT LOSS: On all the Diet Workshop Programs, the average weight loss ranges from one to two pounds per week.

PERSONAL CONSIDERATIONS: The Diet Workshop is on the low end of the cost scale within the industry and offers a variety of different programs. Group sup-port is a key ingredient and clients only pay for the meetings they attend. Additionally, the diet uses gro-cery store food and tries, like Weight Watchers, to try to teach you to eat correctly on your own. If you like the freedom, within certain constraints, to eat what you want, this system might work for you.

On the other hand, if you need a more controlled food plan or hate having to work out all the "units," you might not be happy here. Also, there is less emphasis on exercise here than in other programs even though exercise is a key component to maintaining weight loss over the long term. The Diet Workshop is attempting to deal with this through their new Fitness Walking tape. However, like most other programs, it basically requires you to take full responsibility for starting and maintaining your exercise program.

LOCATION: 30 franchises nationwide primarily in the East Coast, the Midwest, and Florida. Check your Yellow Pages or call or write for specific locations: 10 Brookline Place West, Suite 107-Plaza Level, Brookline, MA 02146 (617) 739-2222.

Formu-3 International

Formu-3 International is a relatively small member of the weight loss industry, one that has taken pains to target smaller communities in the United States. It also features small, mini-centers, which means less overhead and hence lower prices than most other plans. Begun in 1982, it doesn't intend to remain small for long; it has dreams of international (note the name) expansion.

HOW IT WORKS: The Formu-3 system utilizes a grocery store diet built around a list of food exchanges using the four basic food groups. The program is broken down into three phases—weight loss, stabilization, and maintenance.

During the weight loss phase you follow a moderate calorie diet, low in fats, that is based on a relatively wide selection of grocery store food. Throughout this period you visit a personal counselor two to three times per week for support and advice. In addition, Formu-3 provides many suggested menus and recipes based on its food exchange system, to facilitate your shopping and menu planning.

As you approach your goal weight, you shift to the stabilization program which gradually increases your caloric intake until you are neither losing nor gaining weight. When this point is reached, you shift to the maintenance program where the emphasis in meetings with your counselor turns to issues important to keeping the weight off in the long run, such as proper shopping habits, meal planning, strategies for eating out, etc.

THE DIET: Formu-3 refused to give any specifics on its diet.

SUPPLEMENTAL PRODUCTS: Formu-3 does make available optional Formu-Fast foods for purchase by participants in the program. Included are soups, puddings, desserts, and beverages.

STAFF: Staff members all receive training from Formu-3 International headquarters.

COSTS: The price is between $6.90 and $7.65 per week ($398 to $498 for a full year program).

AVERAGE WEIGHT LOSS: Two to three pounds per week.

PERSONAL CONSIDERATIONS: The Formu-3 program is one of the least expensive options around. You should, however, make sure that you can pay on a weekly basis, since different people will require differing lengths of time to get the results they need. As a grocery store based program, it has the benefit of retraining your shopping and food preparation behavior throughout the entire time of the program. Additionally, the individual counseling will be a benefit to those who are uncomfortable in a group or simply too shy to get their needs attended to. However, those who might feel the need of group support would do well to look elsewhere. And it appears to have no exercise component whatsoever, even though exercise is crucial to long-term weight control.

LOCATION: Formu-3 is found predominantly in Ohio and Missouri; however, it is expanding towards the East Coast and the Southwest. You can find the nearest location by writing or calling Formu-3 International, 4790 Douglas Circle N.W., Canton, Ohio 44718 (216) 499-3334.

Michigan Doctors Diet Centers

This program just recently bought out the Quick Weight Loss Center, which had existed throughout Michigan since 1978. It currently has 14 centers but plans to expand in the coming years. The company president is a respected physician in the field of obesity, Dr. Daher Rahi, and the program works through local physicians.

HOW IT WORKS: Michigan Doctors Weight Loss Centers is dedicated to highly individualized weight loss programs. While open to anyone, it specializes in diet programs for those with medical problems such as diabetes and cardiac disease.

When you enroll, you must complete a comprehensive history that includes not only your medical history, but your food history from birth. The survey is meant to elicit specific information about lifelong eating habits to enable the staff to better pinpoint areas of concern. Complete blood tests can also be done for a nominal fee in order to help identify any possible problems.

Your chart is then referred to a medical director, a physician well trained in nutrition, who prescribes a diet based on your individual needs. You then meet with a dietitian to review the plan and a first week of menus is developed.

You are assigned a diet counselor and may visit or call that person as much as you want without incurring additional costs; however, for the first two weeks, the program requires participants to visit their counselors on a daily basis. You are also given complete nutritional information in a small class setting where you can ask questions as well as participate in discussions. The information sessions take place during the first weeks of the program and you may attend as many sessions as you desire.

After the weight loss phase, you are required to participate in the maintenance program for at least one year to assure that the weight that came off stays off. During this period, you continue to have unrestricted access to the program staff to answer any questions.

THE DIET: The diet varies with each individual as to number of calories and kinds of food. The program does not sell food or products, and structures its diets so that individuals do their own shopping at grocery stores.

SUPPLEMENTAL PRODUCTS: None.

STAFF: Nurses, both LPNs and RNs, behavior modification specialists (many with psychology degrees), physicians.

COSTS: $200 to $500 for a full year program, depending on the amount of weight loss necessary. This includes mandatory stabilization and maintenance periods.

AVERAGE WEIGHT LOSS: Will vary depending on the diet prescribed.

PERSONAL CONSIDERATIONS: This system allows you a highly individualized program and unlimited access to the staff without any additional cost. Since you prepare your own meals, presumably the transition to a regular diet will not be too difficult. This program will obviously require a commitment of both time and determination because it lacks the convenience of instant calorie counting systems; on the other hand, it does provides virtually unlimited personal assistance. And the fact that it is physician based should provide some security for those with a need for medical monitoring.

On the down side, like most other programs, the exercise component of this system appears to consist largely of encouragement and some education; the rest is up to you.]

LOCATION: As the name implies, these centers are only located in Michigan. Centers can be found in the Yellow Pages or by contacting the corporate headquarters at 15565 Northland Dr., South Field, Michigan 48075 (313) 559-7386.

Physicians Weight Loss Centers

The headquarters for the Physicians Weight Loss Centers is one of only two programs that refused to provide information. So unfortunately, I was forced to use only the information available in their sales materials. Therefore there are unavoidable pieces missing from this entry. I apologize for any inconvenience.

HOW IT WORKS: This system uses grocery store food and custom tailored diets. It begins with a physical screening including blood chemistry profile, electrocardiogram, and a consultation and evaluation by a physician. Then you start what they call the "Success Plan," in which you cut down on snacks, carefully chart what you've eaten on a food list, and visit the Center daily to be weighed and have your food list reviewed.

After the Success Plan is completed, you begin the Success Plan Diet which is followed for 14 days; then you switch over to the Body Select Diet. You're monitored five days per week during the first two weeks and three days per week thereafter.

You remain on the Body Select Diet until reaching your goal weight, and are then encouraged to enroll in the Weight Maintenance Program. Here you gradually increase your calorie intake to the amount required to maintain your weight given your height and activity level. Also during this period you learn techniques to help stay at your goal weight.

While on the diets, you are introduced to a walking exercise program, attend behavioral modification classes, and receive informal counseling.

THE DIET: The diet is based on teaching dieters to use grocery store food in a healthy and intelligent fashion. To accomplish this, you begin with a 14-day progression of increasingly varied food choices on the Success Plan. You then switch over to the Body Select Diet series that increases allowable calories and provides more options from the food list categories. An example of one day's menus under the Body Select Plan follows:

Breakfast: 1/2 cup high-fiber cereal, 1 cup skim milk, 1 1/2 oranges.

Lunch: 1 Nutritional Supplement, 1 cup lettuce with diet salad dressing, 1 large tomato, 1/2 slice whole wheat bread, 5 large black olives, 1 small pear.

Dinner: 1 Nutritional Supplement, 1 cup lettuce with diet salad dressing, 3 oz. salmon, 1/2 cup cooked asparagus, 1 Crave Savers High-Fiber Cookie, 1/2 cup red raspberries.

SUPPLEMENTAL PRODUCTS: The Physicians Weight Loss Centers offers a number of additional products including a cookbook with meals designed specifically for the diet; nutritional supplements in the form of soups, drinks, puddings and shakes to help provide the protein you need during the diet; salad dressings; high-fiber cookies; and a variety of optional portion-controlled entrees from chicken to beef to pasta. They also offer two audio tape programs focusing on self improvement and a walking exercise program.

STAFF: Physician involvement in monitoring health, nurses, and counselors who are frequently graduates of the program.

COSTS: Approximately $120 to $250 for the Weight Loss phase.

AVERAGE WEIGHT LOSS: Three pounds per week.

PERSONAL CONSIDERATIONS: This program appears to offer a fair degree of individual tailoring of a diet and a considerable degree of staff attention, particularly during the reducing phase. However, without complete information from the program, it is difficult to be comprehensive. It is also difficult to determine whether the lack of cooperation I received is indicative of the attitude of one individual in a leadership position or of the program itself. If you are interested in this system, I strongly suggest following up for further information.

LOCATION: Available in the Midwest and portions of the South. Contact corporate headquarters at 395 Springside Dr., Akron, OH 44443 (800) 322-7952 for the location of a Center nearest you.

Weight Watchers

One of the largest programs in the industry, Weight Watchers is also one of the oldest weight loss plans in the U.S. It was founded in New York in 1963 by Jean Neidich after she had managed to overcome her own weight problem and wanted to help her friends lose weight. Once she got serious about the program as a business, she became affiliated with noted obesity specialist Dr. George Christakis and the program underwent certain changes. In 1983, Weight Watchers was purchased by Heinz (of ketchup fame) and is now available in 52 countries.

HOW IT WORKS: Weight Watchers calls its system the Personal Choice Weight Loss Program. Its goal is to provide a nutritiously sound food plan, teach clients healthy eating habits, encourage a regular exercise program, and provide the support of others who share the same weight loss concerns. Registration can be done at any Weight Watchers meeting or anytime by dropping in at the Center. New registrants are weighed in and sent to an orientation class that explains the overall program.

Weight Watchers offers two plans, Traditional Group Service and the At Work Program. Some Weight Watchers franchises also offer a program called the Inner Circle Service that provides even more personal attention.

Traditional Group Service: With this plan, you attend weekly meetings as often or infrequently as you desire. At the meeting you are weighed in and your weight is recorded in your personal diary. While you may attend as regularly or irregularly as you desire, the program is built around a five-week plan.

The first week you are introduced to the program

and learn how the food exchange lists and daily and weekly food diaries are to be used.

The second week adds additional calories and optional foods, and introduces the Weight Watchers exercise program. Weight Watchers encourages you to check with your doctor regarding any potential issues that might affect your participation in both the diet and the exercise plan, but it also provides a brief Exercise Readiness Quiz designed to pinpoint any potential health problems that would necessitate consultation with your doctor.

The exercise program itself is divided into four levels of increasingly more challenging physical activity and includes numerous options within each level, including walking, jogging, swimming, or bicycling. The exercise plan is designed to bring even the most sedentary folks into a more healthy regime of physical activity and begins with a brief Personal Activity Profile that places you in an appropriate activity level.

Week three adds more foods to the list of acceptable options and opens up the option of restaurant dining. Week four adds additional food options and introduces the Self-Discovery Plan that starts with a Self-Discovery Profile to help you identify the weight loss skills you need. The plan is structured so that you begin working on mastering skills that are relatively simple for you and proceed to more difficult tasks as your confidence builds.

Week five adds more food options, increases your calorie intake to around 1200, and sets you on the course that you will maintain until you reach your desired weight. After that, you attend as many or as few meetings as you want.

The At Work Program: Designed to fit into the workplace and be held on the employer's location, this option is built around the same basics as the Traditional Group Service. However, it emphasizes issues of concern to working people, including business lunches, stress, and cafeteria food.

THE DIET: The diet is built around a system of exchanges. One exchange in any given food group will equal the same number of calories as any other exchange from that food group. There are six different food exchange categories–Fruit, Vegetables, Fat, Protein, Bread, Milk–a seventh floating category from which you can borrow exchanges to meet your personal preferences.

For example, a man or a women in the first week of the diet would eat the following number of exchanges each day:

Exchanges	Men	Women
Fruit	3	2
Vegetables	3	3
Fat	3 to 4	2 to 3
Protein	6 to 7	4 to 5
Bread	4 to 5	2 to 3
Milk	2	2
Floating	1	1

Here's some examples of the kinds and quantities of foods available and what each exchange represents:
Fruit:
  1 small apple
  1 small orange
  1/2 cup orange juice
  1 cup of strawberries
Vegetables (1/2 cup):
  broccoli
  carrots
  green beans

cucumbers
onions
lettuce
tomatoes

Fat:

1 tsp. margarine
1 tsp. mayonnaise
1 tsp. vegetable oil
1 tsp. peanut butter
1 1/2 tsp. salad dressing

Protein:

1 oz. lean beef
1 oz. hard cheese
1 oz. lean pork
1 oz. chicken
1 egg

Bread:

1 slice bread
3/4 oz. cold cereal
1/2 cup cooked pasta
3 oz. potato

Milk:

1 cup skim or nonfat
1/2 cup low-fat yogurt

Optional 10-calorie foods include:

1 tsp. bread crumbs
1 tsp. grated cheese
1/4 cup broth
1/2 tsp. honey

How would all those exchange rates come together into a day's meals? Here's an example:

Breakfast:

1/2 cup strawberries
3/4 oz. cold cereal
1 cup skim milk

Lunch:
    Roast beef sandwich (2 oz. beef, 3 tomato slices,
    lettuce, 1 tsp. mustard and 2 slices of bread)
    6 carrot sticks
Dinner:
    Broiled chicken with garlic sauce
    3 oz. baked potato with 1 tsp. margarine
    4 broccoli spears
    10 grapes
Snacks:
    1 small orange
    1 cup skim milk

In addition to the exchange limits, Weight Watchers restricts the number of certain selections each week. For example, while you have four to seven protein exchanges each day during the first week, you must limit your weekly consumption of eggs to a maximum of three.

All this might appear a little difficult to keep track of, but Weight Watchers makes it easier with a weekly diary that includes a complete list of available food exchanges, suggested menus, recipes complete with exchange totals, and a daily checklist to keep track of exchanges. You even get a Dining Out Guide that translates common menu items into food exchanges.

During the reducing phase of the diet, which begins with 1000 calories, you add additional foods and more optional calories each week. By the fifth week the diet is up to approximately 1200 calories and includes options such as wine, beer, butter, and cookies. You remain at this level until you reach your goal weight.

At that point you shift to the six-week-long Maintenance Plan in which you gradually add exchanges and calories while carefully tracking your weight to determine the level of calories needed to maintain your goal weight. During this time, you continue to attend weekly meetings and work on the skills necessary to keep the weight from returning.

For those who need more structure or would prefer the convenience, Weight Watchers has just introduced what it calls a Personal Cuisine Option. This includes a wide variety of pre-packaged foods that correspond to its system of exchanges. One benefit of this option is that it can be selected on any given week, so you can combine grocery store food and pre-packaged food to suit your own budget, schedule, and inclination. For now, the Personal Cuisine Option is only available in Northern California but there are plans to expand if it is successful.

SUPPLEMENTAL PRODUCTS: In addition to its well-known line of frozen foods, Weight Watchers offers a wide variety of products including cookbooks, an Exchange Manager to keep track of daily exchanges, a engagement calendar, two different fitness book/tape combinations, a variety of scales for accurate portion control, and a monthly magazine.

STAFF: Group leaders are chosen from successful Weight Watcher graduates. They must take a three-month training program and meet monthly with their area supervisor as well as attend an annual meeting.

COSTS: Registration and the first session costs an average of $30 and each meeting attended thereafter is approximately $10.

AVERAGE WEIGHT LOSS: One to two pounds per week.

PERSONAL CONSIDERATIONS: Weight Watchers is one of the least expensive programs available. It does not require packaged food or drinks. It emphasizes learning how to eat for the rest of your life, supporting weight loss at a moderate rate rather than rapidly. Essentially, it teaches you how to change your eating habits, gives you the tools to do it, and provides some weekly support. The rest is up to you.

The overriding theory is that by slowly and surely changing your eating habits, practicing those changes week in and week out at both the grocery store and the dining table, you will arrive ultimately at a weight you can maintain with little effort. Many people really thrive on such a "re-education."

If, however, you feel like you need more personal attention or a more structured situation, or that the moderate rate of weight loss would be too discouraging, this may not be the program for you. Additionally, Weight Watchers does require a fair amount of your time and energy and if convenience is what you are after this is probably not the best option.

LOCATION: Weight Watchers is available around the world. For the location nearest you call (800) 333-3000, write Weight Watchers International, Inc., Jericho Atrium, 500 North Broadway, Jericho, NY 11753, or check your local Yellow Pages.

Packaged Food Programs

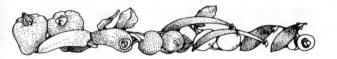

Diet Ease

A relative small fry in the industry, Diet Ease has been in existence for eight years and currently operates approximately 30 centers throughout northern California. It emphasizes convenience and locally-grown frozen food. The hallmark of the program appears to be simplicity.

HOW IT WORKS: The Diet Ease system begins with a determination of your goal weight. You are then placed on the Diet Ease diet and visit the Center on a weekly basis to select and pick up the next week's supply of food. You also meet weekly for 15 to 30 minutes with your individual counselor whose job it is to give you the help and information necessary to successfully complete the program. (You can also call in at any time to get answers to questions you might have regarding the program.) Counselors stress portion control and establishing new eating habits rather than reliance on weighing and measuring foods.

Once you reach your goal weight, you shift to the Trim For Life Program for anywhere from six months to one year. During this phase you continue visits to your Counselor, where you are given one on one help with successfully maintaining your weight loss. Throughout the Trim For Life Program, you may purchase Diet Ease foods as a convenient backup, but are strongly encouraged to rely on grocery store food.

THE DIET: The Diet Ease diet consists of a selection of frozen foods provided through the Centers which are balanced to provide for all your nutritional needs while keeping the caloric count to around 950 calories per day.

Breakfast choices include an assortment of muffins, strudels, a breakfast bar, and breakfast loaves that come frozen and are heated before serving.

Lunches can be selected from 29 possibilities including Pasta Primavera, Spicy Burrito Pocket, Homemade Chili, Beef Stew, Veal with Sage and Cheese Pizza.

Dinner selection include among the 29 selections, a Garden Quiche, Cheese Enchiladas, Manicotti, Lasagna, Chicken Curry, Corn Beef and Cabbage and Veal Parmigiana. You are also allowed two to three cups of fresh or frozen vegetables per day and one selection of fruit.

SUPPLEMENTAL PRODUCTS: None.

STAFF: All staff members go through a training program.

COST: The reducing and maintenance phases combined goes for around $250. Diet Ease food products cost around $66 per week.

AVERAGE WEIGHT LOSS: Two to five pounds per week.

PERSONAL CONSIDERATIONS: Diet Ease stresses convenience and tasty meals and provides this with a weekly package of frozen food that only need to be heated. Most packaged food programs have the disadvantage of not preparing you for the shopping and food preparation that you will need to do after you have lost weight. The Diet Ease theory is that since their program uses fresh frozen food and utilizes local, seasonal food rather than dehydrated food, it will help to re-train your eating habits in a way that you can easily adapt to. However, you still aren't getting the shopping and cooking practice you will ultimately need. Also, the food prices are a bit steep, but again remember you have to adjust that cost by the amount you would use at the grocery store.

One other consideration is that the program appears to be on the casual side relative to counseling, education, exercise, and support. Folks who know they are going to need a very structured approach might do well with another plan.

LOCATION: Available throughout Northern California. Check the Yellow Pages or contact Diet Ease, 14393 E.14th St., Suite 203, San Leandro, CA 94577 (415) 895-5909.

Jenny Craig Weight Loss Centres

The Jenny Craig method can be traced back to Jenny Craig herself; the foundation of the program was developed over 30 years ago as she struggled with her own excessive weight gain after her second pregnancy. In 1970 she went to work at Body Contour Inc., a growing weight loss company that her soon-to-be husband Sid Craig ran. After 12 years and over 200 weight-loss centers, Sid and Jenny Craig had a disagreement with their partners over the proper direction to take. As a result, in 1982 the Body Contour Centers were sold, ironically to what would soon be one of their largest competitors–Nutri/System.

Since they had promised not to compete in the domestic weight loss industry for two years, Sid and Jenny immediately moved to Australia and opened their first Jenny Craig Weight Loss Centre. By 1985 the no-competition agreement with Nutri/System had expired, and the company began an expansion that continues today. It now has over 500 Centres in the United States, Canada, Puerto Rico, New Zealand, Australia, and Great Britain.

HOW IT WORKS: The system has three components: exercise, lifestyle changes, and light meals consisting of Jenny Craig packaged foods. It includes two weekly visits to the center: one with an individual counselor and one with a group. Upon enrollment, you must fill out a health questionnaire and if you have specific health problems, must get a doctor's written permission before beginning.

At the first visit, you spend 20 minutes with a weight loss counselor where with the assistance of a computer you establish your goal weight. At subsequent private visits, your counselor focuses on setting specific exercise and behavioral change goals, goes over the progress and problems of the prior week, weighs you in, and gets your menu and packaged foods for the next week. Throughout the program you keep a careful diary that is designed to help you become more aware of your food behavior patterns.

The second visit of the week is to attend a Lifestyle Class with between 12 and 20 other clients and a Lifestyle Class Facilitator. The facilitator uses a series of 17 videotapes on subjects like nutrition, psychology, exercise, etc., to transmit information and to promote group discussion. These include "Why People Eat," "Knowing When to Stop," and "Controlling Binge Eating." Each class concludes with a behavioral assignment to be practiced at home during the week (for example, practicing a time-out procedure to control binge eating). You are also encouraged to make use at home of a series of audio tapes that reinforce class information.

Once you are halfway to your desired weight level, you begin, with the assistance of your counselor, planning your own meals from grocery store food two days a week. This continues until you reach your goal weight. At that point, you enter the Permanent Stabilization Program which runs for one year. During this time you may continue to purchase Jenny Craig cuisine, see your counselor and attend LifeStyle Classes. Included as a part of the Permanent Stabilization Program are 14

Maintenance Classes that focus on teaching skills to help prevent a relapse into old eating habits.

THE DIET: The Jenny Craig diet is made up of packaged foods you must buy from the Centre, supplemented by certain grocery store items. It contains approximately 1,000 calories per day for women, and 1200 to 1400 calories per day for men.

Individual needs and circumstances are taken into account when planning your diet. However, unlike most other weight loss programs, there is very little flexibility in the daily menus. If a person is strongly adverse to a particular food, an entirely different menu day is substituted; counselors are not allowed simply to substitute for the objectionable food item. By taking this approach, Jenny Craig is certain that minimum nutritional requirements are satisfied.

Here are two sample daily menus:

DAY ONE
Breakfast:
    1 Jenny Craig Banana Bran Muffin
    1/2 cup skim milk
Snack:
    1 orange
Lunch:
    Jenny Craig Minestrone Soup
    4 carrot sticks
Snack:
    2 rice cakes
    low-cal drink
Dinner:
    Jenny Craig Salisbury Steak Champignon with Pota
    toes au Gratin and Green Beans
Snack:
    1 cup plain yogurt
    1 pear

62

DAY TWO
Breakfast:
    1 Jenny Craig Chocolate Drink
    1 slice wheat toast with 1 tsp. margarine
Snack:
    1/2 grapefruit
Lunch:
    1 Jenny Craig Chicken Salad over shredded lettuce
    1 wheat roll with 1 tsp. margarine
    1 apple
Snack:
    1/2 cup plain yogurt
Dinner:
    1 Jenny Craig Cappelletti
    1 cup garden salad with Jenny Craig salad dressing
Snack:
    Jenny Craig Chocolate Mousse

Beginning when you are halfway to your goal weight, grocery store food is re-introduced gradually. Beginning at your goal weight, calories are increased until you reach a level that will maintain your current weight.

SUPPLEMENTAL PRODUCTS: A Jenny Craig Walking Program, two audio casettes and a booklet for beginners through advanced exercisers for $25.

STAFF: Both Lifestyle Facilitators and Weight Loss Counselors receive 48 hours worth of initial training and are required to attend a continuing education class every month. In addition, the head office appoints one trainer/quality assurance person for approximately every four Jenny Craig Centres; it is that person's responsibility to assure that the staff is kept fully apprised of all changes and new information, both about nutrition and Jenny Craig policy, and that the Centre is implementing the program exactly as it was designed.

COSTS: The total package, including weight loss, 12-month weight maintenance program, and the Lifestyle counseling program is approximately $300. The weight loss portion itself can be found for between $79 and $99. The packaged food averages about $60 per week.

AVERAGE WEIGHT LOSS: One to two pounds per week.

PERSONAL CONSIDERATIONS: Jenny Craig believes that using packaged foods is not only convenient, but it retrains clients who have demonstrated an inability to make appropriate food-related decisions. By restricting people to the menus provided, Jenny Craig believes clients master proper portion control, and learn to eat low-sodium and low-fat foods that taste good.

Because the diet is so controlled, however, some people have trouble readjusting to eating their own food, although the program attempts to address this problem by re-introducing grocery store foods halfway through the weight loss. This may not be enough. You should also consider whether you will be able to make the transition from Jenny Craig foods to the grocery store without falling off the weight control wagon. Additionally, the packaged food is not cheap, but you must remember that for each meal you purchase from Jenny Craig you don't have to buy one at the store.

The program also offers a relatively structured support system, with good nutritional information and an exercise component; however, like most of the other diet programs, the exercise program is largely dependant upon your own personal diligence--even though without it, you may have difficulty keeping the lost pounds from returning.

LOCATION: Jenny Craig Centres are found around the world. Corporate headquarters are: 445 Marine View Drive, Suite 300, Del Mar, CA 92014 (619) 259-7000.

The Micro Diet

The Micro Diet, or as the Uni-Vite company is fond of calling it, the "Amazing Micro Diet," was developed in Great Britain in the early 1980s from research breakthrough in Very Low Calorie Diets. After rapid expansion in the British market and the successful expansion of the program to the rest of Europe, Micro Diet has recently come to the United States. With an average of between 630 and 940 calories per day, the Micro Diet tends to include more calories and food choices than most Very Low Calorie Diets, and fewer calories and food choices than more conventional moderate calorie diets. The Micro Diet people themselves split the difference and call it a Low Calorie Diet.

HOW IT WORKS: Based on a system of nutritional food replacements, The Micro Diet Program is distributed through independent "Micro Diet Advisors" who encourage, support, and advise you during your participation in the diet, as well as act as your supplier of Micro Diet products. Additionally, Advisors attempt to put together group support mechanisms in their local areas for those who want the additional assistance provided by a group of committed dieters.

Micro Diet has designed its program to be as flexible as possible, and thus offers a variety of different approaches. The fastest weight loss comes from the Sole Source approach. If you are using Micro Diet products as the sole source of food, you select a daily regime from a chart that explains what combination of Micro Diet foods equals how many calories. You may choose different combinations of the Micro Diet products each day, but the selection must follow the chart in order to ensure you get the proper balance of nutritional elements on any given day. Micro Diet recommends that you not stay on the Sole Source diet for more than three consecutive weeks. If more weight needs to be lost, it advises you spend a week eating a moderate calorie diet of regular food before returning to the Sole Source plan. It also recommends that people beginning a diet should first consult with their physician.

A second option is Sole Source/Fiber Plus approach in which you follow the Micro Diet chart for meal selections, but add to it high fiber options such as fruit and vegetables. This will add calories and decrease the rate of weight loss, but will allow for some directed snacking.

The third approach is called Two Plus One. Here you select two meals per day from the Micro Diet products and eat a third regular meal. Once again this will obviously add calories but will also allow for the option of eating the same food as family members.

The Combo Plan involves following the Sole Source diet during the week and shifting to Two Plus One on the weekends. This is designed to allow for continued dieting without intruding into weekend socializing. Alternately, you may simply choose on a day-to-day basis which plan to follow.

The Micro Diet also comes with a copy of the book, *The Amazing Micro Diet* (1985), that details the origins of the program, contains basic information regarding diet and exercise, includes a section on how to keep the pounds off after the diet, and is sprinkled with testimonial case studies of successful dieters. The book also contains a variety of recipes to vary the taste of Micro Diet products.

THE DIET: The program is based on a mix and match selection of Micro Diet low calorie products that include shakes (in Chocolate, Strawberry, Vanilla and Tropical Orange flavors) that are designed to be mixed with water or other non-caloric beverages; 2.75-ounce meal bars in Peanut, Cinnamon and Chocolate; soups in either Vegetable or Chicken flavor; Muesli, and Chili.

The Micro drinks, Chili, and soups all contain 210 calories per serving. Both the Peanut and Cinnamon bars equal 260 calories while the Chocolate bar, as chocolate will do, adds a few extra calories to total 295 calories. The Muesli is a high fiber cereal mix that includes oat flakes, soy, currants, peanuts, and wheat flakes and totals 260 calories.

Each product is formulated to be high in nutritional content so that when eaten in pre-selected combinations, you receive 100 percent of Recommended Daily Allowances. When taken according to the selection chart the Micro Diet consists of approximately 53 percent carbohydrates, 43 percent protein and 6 percent fat.

The selection chart provides 14 different daily meal options from a lowest calorie count of 630 for two shakes and soup, to the highest calorie selection of 940 calories for one shake, one soup, one peanut or cinnamon bar, and a bowl of Muesli.

If you select an approach other than Sole Source, your daily calorie intake will differ depending upon what other foods you eat.

SUPPLEMENTAL PRODUCTS: Micro Diet sells *The Shape-Up Video* by Jackie Genova. It includes a three-part exercise program, "Limber Up" for those just beginning to exercise, "Tone Up" for mid-level activities, and "Shape Up" for those already in fit condition.

STAFF: Micro Diet Advisors are independent distributors. They are given basic instruction in the products and the program but do not have any special training.

COST: Micro Diet offeres a special introductory package of 20 meals for $39.95. Their regular prices are around $2.00 per meal. Videos are approximately $12-$15.

AVERAGE WEIGHT LOSS: Will vary depending upon how the program is used, but should range from one to four pounds per week.

PERSONAL CONSIDERATIONS: While the Micro Diet people stress the importance of your Micro Diet Advisor, it is probably wise to consider this a essentially self-operating program where the bulk of the structure, motivation, and discipline will be your responsibility. If you know what you want to achieve and feel comfortable in controlling your own progress, there is considerable flexibility available. However, if you feel that left to your own devices you are more apt to stray from the program you might consider a more structured approach.

Micro Diet does a better job on the exercise component than most systems, offering a progressive video; however you must rely on personal motivation to carry through with the plan.

Additionally the Sole Source program provides rapid weight loss with a greater variety of meal replacement options than many other programs and Micro Diet products are priced relatively inexpensively compared with other Very Low Calorie Diet programs (remember, as with all meal replacement programs you need to consider the money you will save at the grocery store in evaluating the ultimate cost of the program). However, if you are considering this option, you should realize that, according to most definitions, the Sole Source approach would qualify as a Very Low Calorie Diet. You should read the chapter in this book regarding VLCDs and definitely consult your physician before beginning.

One other possible disadvantage is that while you are eating Micro Diet products you don't get much practice in everyday healthy food selection. Nor do you get much help in basic nutritional re-education. Therefore the transition back to grocery store food may be more difficult, and there might be a temptation to rely on Micro Diet products well beyond the weight loss phase as a hedge against regaining weight.

LOCATION: Available nationwide. Check your Yellow Pages or contact Uni-Vite Inc., 2440 Impala Dr., Carlsbad CA 92008 (619) 931-9942.

Nutri/System

Nutri/System is the giant of the weight loss industry. Established in 1971 in Philadelphia, it has grown to international proportions with over 1,700 centers throughout the United States, Canada, Australia, and the United Kingdom. As of 1990 Nutri/System was serving more than 200,000 clients per week.

HOW IT WORKS: The program is designed around a system of packaged food, exercise, and support groups. Upon signing up, you are given a tour of the local center and interviewed by a weight consultant about eating habits, weight history, lifestyle, and activity level. You must also fill out a health history and a Personalized Weight Loss Profile Questionnaire that is designed to uncover obstacles that might arise during the program. For example, it will alert the staff to those who are particularly shy and the Nutri/System folks will then go out of their way to introduce that person to others in the support group.

With the information provided, a staff person then prints out a computer-generated analysis based on the Metropolitan Life Insurance table for ideal weight while taking into consideration age, gender, how much weight you need to lose, and other personal considerations. This analysis also establishes a weight goal and a timetable for reaching that goal. You then meet your Nutritional Specialist, are introduced to the appropriate Nutri/System CRAVE FREE meal plan, and helped to fill out your weekly meal plan. Subsequently you have weekly one-on-one weigh-ins with your Nutritional Specialist, where you discuss any problems, ask questions, and go over the next week's meal plan. These meetings usually last ten minutes or so and then you go to a small group discussion (usually six to eight people) led by a Behavior Breakthrough Counselor. These meetings usually last around a half hour and stress modifying eating habits and dealing with specific problems through group inter-action and personal attention. Clients are also provided at-home study materials as necessary on specific issues.

In the third week you are introduced to the Body Breakthrough Activity Plan. This home exercise pro-gram was designed to provide a selection of activities broken down into a three-part program. The first phase involves making changes in every day activities in order to give your metabolic rate a boost. These can be as simple as parking farther away from your destination and walking part of the way, or getting off the bus one stop before home to walk the rest of the way. Phase two involves a walking program that starts gradually, and the third phase includes videos on three separate levels of low-impact aerobic exercises.

After reaching a healthy weight, you enter the main-tenance program with continued weekly meetings with the Nutritional Specialist, who helps you make the transition from packaged food to grocery store food. For example, when approaching your goal weight, you will begin meal planning and using an exchange system. Group sessions will change focus as well; there are now classes on how to shop at the grocery store and how to read food labels.

At this point you cut back your use of Nutri/System food to only two days per week, while continuing sessions with your Counselor once a week for six months, then once every two weeks for the next three months and then finally once a month for three months. Throughout this period you can go more often if necessary. Additionally, you continue meeting weekly with your Behavior Breakthrough Classes with a new emphasis on issues specific to keeping the lost pounds from returning.

Nutri/System offers a special rebate to those who successfully keep weight off in the maintenance program. In order to qualify, you must have kept up with the program and kept within five pounds of your goal weight.

THE DIET: The "Crave-Free" diet consists of packaged foods that are purchased through Nutri/System. Each item has a specific calorie and nutritional content so that by following the plan dieters will receive proper nutrition while controlling calorie intake. You are given considerable leeway in the choice of food, and if you have any particular allergies or health problems your counselor can always call the home office directly to have a diet tailored to your personal needs.

The basic diet meets all the U.S. RDA standards, contains around 1000 to 1100 calories per day, and consists of 61 percent carbohydrates, 25 percent protein and 14 percent fat. Nutri/System also has a 1200 and 1500 calorie diet for those who need more calories per day, and has specially modified diets for people who are lactose controlled, aspartame sensitive, hypoglycemic, or vegetarian.

Breakfast includes one entree such as Oat Bran Flakes Cereal, Oatmeal Cereal, Toasted Grains Cereal, or Pancakes or Waffles with Syrup. Also included in the breakfast menu is a four-ounce glass of skim milk, two eight-ounce glasses of water, ice tea, or Orange Citrus beverage. For a morning snack, dieters may have a hot drink such as the Nutri/System Cinnamon Coffee or Cocoa and a diet beverage.

Lunch consists of one entree like a beef taco, salami, ham or cheese slices, chicken noodle or cream of chicken soup, plus a salad with salad dressing, rolls or crackers, and dietetic beverages. The afternoon snack is selected from "Craving Control" snacks such as Chocolate Flavor Chews, Fruit Flavor Chews, Microwave Popcorn, Sesame Pretzels, and Nacho Flavor Crisps.

Dinner includes an entree selected from a list of over 25 options like Beef with Green Peppers and Onions, Chili Dog, Cheese Ravioli, Lasagna, and Spaghetti with Meatballs. You also eat one cup of any selected vegetable from a list of around 30 options, one Nutri/System dessert like caramel popcorn, Chocolate Chip Cookie Apple Cinnamon Cupcakes, or Orange Sherbet. For an evening snack you choose again from the selection of "Craving Control" snacks.

With each meal you drink either a glass of water or a Nutri/System Ice Tea or Orange Citrus Drink.

SUPPLEMENTAL PRODUCTS: Nutri/System offers a cookbook.

STAFF: All Nutri/System staff members go through a three-month training program at Nutri/System University. Behavior Breakthrough Counselors may or may not have a psychological background, but all are trained by the Nutri/System head office.

COSTS: Like most programs, Nutri/System offers frequent specials and the prices will vary from location to location. However, a program designed to lose 30 pounds would run around $600 and Nutri/System foods run approximately $65 per week.

Individuals who faithfully comply with the program and do not reach their goal weight within the established timetable continue to receive all the services of the Nutri/System program free until their goal weight is reached; they must pay, however, for food they use.

AVERAGE WEIGHT LOSS: One and a half to two pounds per week.

PERSONAL CONSIDERATIONS: The Nutri/System diet relies on packaged foods that you pick up once a week. For people who are leading busy lives and don't want to worry about counting calories and measuring portions, this can be a real benefit. The program is also fairly structured, with support systems in place to help you over the rough spots, some sound re-education efforts, and an exercise component, which essentially relies on you to folllow through on your own. But at least there is some emphasis placed on teaching and encouraging active exercise.

A disadvantage to some folks, however, will be the same thing that is a plus for others–the packaged food. You must be willing to live within the limited variety available. And, since during most of the reducing phase of the program you are not shopping at the grocery store, those who love cooking may find it less than enjoyable or convenient. Additionally, as with all packaged food plans, you may have trouble making the transition back to home-prepared food.

Another possible problem is that while Nutri/System packaged foods present some interesting choices such as tacos, chocolate chip cookies, and salami, they are not the best of examples for a dieter. For when you are off Nutri/System food, you may gain weight eating such items found in the grocery store; it is unlikely that Nutri/System chocolate chip cookies have the same number of calories as the chocolate chip cookies in the grocery store.

Finally, because of the cost of the packaged food, this plan may simply be too expensive, although you must remember for comparison purposes to discount the price by the amount you would usually spend at the grocery store.

LOCATION: Available nationwide. Check the Yellow Pages or contact corporate headquarters at 3901 Commerce Ave., Suite 925, Willow Grove, PA 19090 (800) 321 8446.

Very Low Calorie Diets

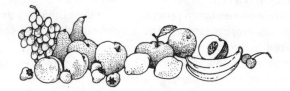

Health Management Resources
(HMR)

HMR is one of the largest providers of Very Low Calorie Diet meal replacement programs in the country. It operates out of hospitals and other medical settings; its original program is designed to serve those who are at least 20 percent overweight or need to lose over 40 pounds. It has recently added a program that does not require close medical supervision for those with less than 40 pounds to lose and no medical problems.

HOW IT WORKS: The plan begins with a free pre-registration orientation program where the outlines of the program are presented. Those interested then fill out an application form and a complete health history. You are then given an appointment for an initial clinical evaluation where you undergo a complete physical, with all appropriate blood and urine tests as well as an EKG.

Medically Supervised Program: The regular program is a Very Low Calorie Diet that requires complete abstinence from grocery store food during which all your calories and nutritional requirements are satisfied through a formula replacement.

This program run 14 to 16 weeks during the weight loss phase or longer if necessary to reach your goal weight. Throughout this period, you are medically monitored each week and are required to attend weekly small group educational sessions. These sessions stress sound nutritional principles, the need for an active exercise program, and the assistance needed to help you through the diet.

Once you approach your goal weight, you enter the re-feeding phase where grocery store food is gradually reintroduced into your diet as you are weaned from the food replacement formulas. During this period, which run between four and six weeks, you continue to attend weekly group sessions; the focus shifts to reinforcing the skills necessary to maintain your weight loss once back on a grocery store diet.

HMR has developed its own calorie evaluation system designed to help you accurately estimate the calories in just about any food without having to refer to calorie charts. With this system, you are taught a program of calorie balancing that allows you to eat any foods you want by consciously balancing your calorie intake.

After the re-feeding phase you enter the Maintenance Program which last a full 18 months. During this period, you continue to attend weekly group meetings to help you develop long term food behavior patterns that will allow you to eat a balanced diet without regaining the weight you lost.

The Medically Unsupervised Program: This program runs approximately ten weeks, and follows the basic outlines of the Medically Supervised Program, complete with weekly group meetings and individual help; the only exception is that you are not required to visit a physician each week. Additionally, during the reducing phase of the unsupervised program, you eat two meals per day of HMR's pre-packaged foods, and use the HMR nutritional formulas to supplement those two meals. The maintenance phase for the medically unsupervised program runs six months.

THE DIET: The HMR diet is built around very low calorie nutritional formulas: HMR 500 (520 calories per day) and HMR 800 (800 calories per day. When taken as complete meal replacements, both formulas supply more than 100 percent of your U.S. RDA.

New to the program are pre-packaged entrees now

available for both the medically supervised and unsupervised program. These include: Chicken Breast with Mushroom Sauce and Beef Lentil Soup with Vegetables at 150 calories per entree; Chicken Stew, Seven-Bean Soup, Chicken Gumbo, and Shrimp and Rice with Tomato Sauce at 170 calories per entree; Turkey Chili with Beans and Pasta with Tomato Sauce at 200 calories per entree; and Chicken and Rice with Tomato Sauce at 230 calories per entree.

SUPPLEMENTAL PRODUCTS: None.

STAFF: HMR centers are staffed by physicians, nurses, registered dietitians, psychologists, and other health care professionals.

COSTS: The Medically Supervised Program runs approximately $2300 inclusive of medical exams, tests, etc. as well as all entrees and nutritional formulas for the reducing and re-feeding portion of the plan and an additional $990 for the 18-month maintenance phase.

The Medically Unsupervised Program is approximately $1170 inclusive for the reducing and re-feeding phase, and an additional $330 for the maintenance phase.

AVERAGE WEIGHT LOSS: Two to five pounds per week.

PERSONAL CONSIDERATIONS: The HMR Medically Supervised Program is one of the most highly-structured programs available, although like virtually all programs, does not offer a monitored exercise program. It is a Very Low Calorie Diet and you should read the chapter on those diets carefully and consult your own doctor before making a decision. It also includes the longest mandatory maintenance period (18 months). The obvious benefit of this is that your potential chance for long term success is greater than with a plan with a shorter maintenance time. HMR also provides an obvious benefit for those people with medical problems that require close monitoring.

The unsupervised program is a kind of hybrid between meal replacement formula systems and pre-packaged food plans. As such, it has the disadvantage of not providing much hands-on retraining in shopping and cooking during the weight loss period. However, this may be somewhat compensated for by the length of the maintenance program. Both programs are relatively expensive, but do provide very highly trained professional staffs to assist you.

LOCATION: Nationwide. You can find the one nearest you by writing or calling Health Management Resources, 59 Temple Place, Suite 704, Boston MA 02111 (617) 357-9876.

Metabolic Nutrition Program

The Metabolic Nutrition Program was developed in 1982 by the Contra Costa Endocrine Associates based in Walnut Creek, CA. It is a physician-based program targeted at patients who need to lose 40 pounds or more in order to attain a healthy weight. The program is supervision intensive and stresses long-term program involvement (up to one to two years) in order to promote lifetime maintenance of healthy weight levels.

HOW IT WORKS: This is a highly structured, Very Low Calorie Diet that uses a modified fast during which you consume only pre-packaged liquid supplements. Participants in the program must first attend a free orientation program where they are introduced to the basics. If you decide to join the program, you are given a physical examination including an electrocardiogram and a battery of laboratory tests to evaluate potential health risks and determine a goal weight in consultation with a physician.

Phase One, The Protein Sparing Modified Fast: During this phase, you are put on a strict 605 calorie-per-day diet of MNP 70/70, a liquid dietary supplement that is consumed five times per day. Vitamin supplements, included in the cost of the program, are taken daily, and you are examined by a physician each week and receive biweekly laboratory tests. Additionally, you are provided with informational weight control aids, encouraged to begin a regular exercise program and are given homework assignments such as wearing a pedometer to keep track of the miles you walk, or going to the store to purchase five dollars worth of your favorite food to throw away as a graphic and dramatic demonstration that "wasting" small amounts of food is not the end of the world, and you don't have to eat every bite of food placed in front of you.

You must also participate in small group psychological counseling sessions. The program offers the choice of task-oriented sessions that focus on eating habits and weight control, or in-depth psychotherapy that deals with psychological factors involved in weight control. You remain on the MNP 70/70 supplement until the goal weight is reached.

Phase Two, Transition: This period last four weeks, and real food is gradually introduced as you are weaned from the MNP 70/70 supplement. Diet changes take place weekly after a meeting with the dietitian; during the first week, a solid protein is introduced and one complete meal is then added each subsequent week.

Weekly group therapy sessions continue with an emphasis on adjusting eating behavior, nutritional education, and lifestyle changes. Additionally, you continue to see the physician weekly and have biweekly laboratory tests.

Phase Three, Maintenance: Participants are requested to contract to maintain a reasonable weight range over six months and to continue with therapy sessions throughout this period. During this time, you attend monthly hands-on group nutrition sessions such as going to the supermarket en mass and reading labels. Another session might include a low-calorie salad dressing taste test. You also meet monthly on an individual basis with a dietitian and are examined by a physician every four weeks.

After the six-month maintenance period is completed, you are encouraged to stay with the program for up to one to two years in order to assure that new eating and lifestyle habits become firmly entrenched.

THE DIET: During the weight loss phase of the program, the diet consists solely of the prepackaged liquid MNP 70/70 supplement. Mixed with water or other non-caloric beverages, it comes in chocolate, vanilla, lactose-free vanilla, strawberry, and chicken. The 70/70 refers to its base composition of 70 grams of protein and 70 grams of carbohydrates. The supplement is combined with vitamin and mineral tablets so that you receive 100 percent of RDA.

During the transition and maintenance phase you are instructed in which foods to choose from, taught how to count calories, and helped along with individual assistance from the dietitian. However, diet selection and control is up to you.

SUPPLEMENTAL PRODUCTS: The Metabolic Nutrition Program does not sell any additional products; however it has designed its own computer program for monitoring patient health during participation in the program. Some long-term benefits can be anticipated from this approach as statistical information is accumulated relative to the effects of Very Low Calorie Diets on different health factors.

STAFF: Physician based, the plan includes regular medical exams and laboratory testing. Group therapy sessions are staffed by psychologists and the nutritional counselors are all registered dietitians.

COST: Inclusive of all required products and services:
Initial physical exam and lab tests: $260.
Phase I, MNP 70/70 diet: $465 per four-week period.
Phase II, Transition (four weeks): $425.
Phase III, Maintenance (six months): $485.

Patients who successfully complete maintenance program receive a $120 rebate.

AVERAGE WEIGHT LOSS: Women lose approximately three pounds per week and men lose approximately five pounds per week in Phase I.

PERSONAL CONSIDERATIONS: The Metabolic Nutrition Program is a highly structured program with a number of fairly unique twists. Geared to folks who need to lose a lot of weight, it is one of the only programs that offers the choice between task-oriented and in-depth psychological group therapy.

It suffers from the same problems all Very Low Calorie Diets have in helping you make the transition to better food behavioral choices when the diet itself does not involve food. However, it compensates with an aggressive, hands-on approach to nutritional education. If you've tried other, less structured approaches with little success, perhaps this will work for you. While the program is expensive, remember also when calculating cost comparisons that at least for the reducing phase, you will not be purchasing any food at the store. The Metabolic Nutrition Program is a Very Low Calorie Diet so you should also read the chapter discussing such diets and consult your personal doctor before making any decision.

LOCATION: The Metabolic Nutrition Program currently has 19 centers, four in Texas, one in Chicago, one in Baltimore, one in Pittsfield, MA, and the rest in California. To find the center nearest to you, contact corporate headquarters at 112 La Casa Via, Suite 120, Walnut Creek, CA 94598 (415) 933-3438.

MediBase

The MediBase Program is a medically supervised Very Low Calorie Diet that is only available through hospitals and medical centers. Geared to serve the seriously obese patients, MediBase is a product of Advanced Healthcare and was one of the earliest companies involved in the development and testing of low calorie liquid diets. From its California origins, it has recently begun to spread nationwide.

HOW IT WORKS: The program begins with an initial evaluation period, when you are given a complete medical examination, including a full battery of laboratory tests. Then you are interviewed regarding current food behavioral patterns, and asked to keep an detailed food diary over a five-to-seven-day period that not only lists what was eaten but when it was eaten, where you were, your mood at the time, and if you were in the company of others or not. During this evaluation period, your target weight is established. You are then ready to begin.

Phase I Rapid Weight Loss: During this period you consume nothing but the MediBase formula three times per day. This phase can last from two to six months depending on how much weight you need to lose. By making you break completely with solid foods, the program attempts to stop the bad food behavioral habits of the past and prepare you to learn new and healthier ones. During this phase, you see a staff physician on a biweekly basis for health monitoring and personal counseling, and attend weekly group counseling sessions where you can share your problems with others and are coached on issues such as understanding the risks and benefits of a Very Low Calorie Diet, how to build a support system, understanding the full implications of being overweight, planning an activity program, and understanding your eating behavioral patterns.

Phase II Moderate Weight Loss/Transition Phase: This is a 16-week period during which you are gradually weaned from the MediBase supplement and reintroduced to a healthy food diet. Weight loss continues during the first weeks of this phase and gradually stabilizes around the eighth week. Physician visits are cut back to once every four weeks and the counseling sessions continue on a weekly basis. The focus of the counseling sessions shifts to helping you make the kinds of changes in your food behavior that are necessary for long term success.

Phase III Maintenance Phase: During this phase, you learn how to make intelligent food choices on a daily basis as you prepare menus and meals for the day. The maintenance period can go from 20 weeks to longer, and is designed to reinforce the gains made during the program. You continue to attend group sessions, now on a biweekly basis. The MediBase program places great emphasis on this phase since it is crucial to whether you are able to keep the weight off. To that end, they strongly recommend that you stay involved in the maintenance phase long enough to strengthen and solidify your hopefully new and improved food decisions.

During this phase you are often treated to a wide variety of videotapes and audiovisual demonstrations of different nutritional issues along with the usual group sessions that now focus on the more daily issues of proper food selection, the importance of and practicalities of exercise, and specific health issues.

THE DIET: The MediBase diet consists of a total solid food replacement formula that comes in chocolate, vanilla, and strawberry drinks as well as a chicken soup variation, and is taken three times per day. The formula is slightly different from most of the very low calorie diet formulas on the market. The MediBase formula uses whey protein concentrate and soy protein as its base instead of the usual egg white and milk protein. MediBase believes this provides a more acceptable flavor and texture.

The formula provides 100 percent of the U.S. RDA when taken three times per day, and consists of only 420 calories. It is approximately 45 percent protein (45 grams), 54 percent carbohydrates (54 grams), and 1 percent fat (3 grams).

SUPPLEMENTAL PRODUCTS: None.

STAFF: Staff qualifications differ slightly from location to location; however, the program is physician based, usually found in a hospital or medical clinic, and frequently has both a registered dietitian and a licensed behavioral therapist involved. All staff members, whether professional or not, are trained by MediBase to properly operate the program.

COSTS: The modified program runs approximately $260 per month all inclusive and the full program is around $380 per month all inclusive.

AVERAGE WEIGHT LOSS: Four to five pounds per week.

PERSONAL CONSIDERATIONS: MediBase is a Very Low Calorie Diet and anyone interested should refer to the chapter on Very Low Calorie Diets for more detailed information regarding the history and potential risks of such diets. You should also consult your personal physician.

A very structured program, MediBase shares with all Very Low Calorie Diets the problems inherent in helping you make the transition from no food to changed food habits and behavior. It also shares with most programs the apparent problem of encouraging exercise but leaving it pretty much up to you to get started and keep it up.

LOCATION: MediBase is available nationwide. You can find the program nearest you by contacting Advanced Healthcare, 2801 Salinas Highway, Building F, Monterey, CA 93940 (800) 553-1754.

Medifast

Medifast is a Very Low Calorie Diet designed for those individuals who met the medical definition of obesity—at least 20 percent over their ideal body weight. It was developed in 1972 by one of the pioneers in the field of Very Low Calorie Diets, Dr. William J. Vitale. For a number of years the program was operated out of the Nutrition Institute of Maryland which continues to function as the educational arm for participating physicians. In 1979, Dr. Vitale founded Jason Pharmaceutical and now runs Medifast from there.

HOW IT WORKS: The Medifast program has four phases: Medical Evaluation, Weight Reduction, Realimentation, and Maintenance.

During the Medical Evaluation, you are given a complete medical evaluation including a medical history, urinalysis, blood tests and EKG. Stage two is the reducing phase, where you are placed on a strict regime of five Medifast beverages per day and no other food. Throughout this phase you are monitored on a weekly or biweekly basis by a physician. You also participate in regular meetings of a group called Lifestyle Program of Patient Support where, through a combination of slide presentations and lectures, you deal with such issues as self-esteem, nutrition, relationships, fitness, and healthy living.

Phase three is the gradual reintroduction of solid food. Over a period of time you shift from an exclusive diet of Medifast supplements to a healthy and nutritionally aware use of grocery store food. During this period LifeStyle meetings continue with a renewed emphasis on helping you make the transition back to grocery store food. Finally, the Maintenance phase is devoted to helping you develop the eating, shopping, and behavioral patterns necessary to keep weight off.

THE DIET: The Medifast diet consists of drinking five servings per day of a very low calorie beverage that comes in chocolate, vanilla, strawberry, and orange flavors. Five servings of Medifast 55 for women contain 450 calories, and five servings of Medifast 70 for men contain 480 calories.

SUPPLEMENTAL PRODUCTS: None.

STAFF: Medifast is operated through physicians, hospitals, and medical centers. Staffing will vary with the location.

COSTS: Approximately $1000 to $1200 for a 16-week program.

AVERAGE WEIGHT LOSS: Three to five pounds per day.

PERSONAL CONSIDERATIONS: Medifast is a very structured, physician-based Very Low Calorie Diet so you should read the chapter on very Low Calorie Diets and consult your doctor before making a decision. It is also a complete food replacement program which has the advantage of creating a complete break with regular food habits, but the disadvantage of a more difficult retraining period when you return to eating store food. It does offer group support and behavior modification, but leaves the crucial exercise component of your diet plan up to you to implement and maintain.

While Medifast, like most physician-based programs, is relatively expensive, you should consider that the cost includes all the "food" you will be eating during the reducing phase so you will save some money at the grocery store.

LOCATION: Medifast began in the Mid-Atlantic states and is now available throughout the U.S. Contact Jason Pharmaceuticals, Inc., P.O. Box 370, Owings Mills, MD 21117 (301) 581-8042.

Optifast

Available only through the medical community, Optifast grew out of the working relationship between the Doyle Company and Dr. Victor Vertes of Mt. Sinai Hospital in Cleveland, one of the early developers of liquid protein sparing formulas. The Doyle Company was purchased by Sandoz in 1984, and Optifast emerged to become one of the most widely used of the physician-based programs.

HOW IT WORKS: Optifast is a medically intensive, highly structured program based on the premise that obesity is a chronic disease that, while controllable, will reoccur in the absence of long-term therapy. Optifast patients typically are 50 to 60 percent above their ideal weight, and physicians at Optifast have concluded that in order to lose that much weight, patients must be treated with a combination of a Very Low Calorie Diet, nutritional education, behavioral therapy, and exercise. The program is offered through hospitals and medical centers, and involves a year-long, six-phase timetable.

Phase One is an initial evaluation with one of the Optifast physicians during which you undergo a battery of tests including a complete medical exam, blood tests, medical history, and psychological and nutritional assessments. The nutritional assessment begins with a lengthy questionnaire dealing with eating habits, readiness to diet, stressful situations, exercise habits, etc., and is carefully reviewed by a psychologist. You are also introduced to the food diary, which assists in developing self-awareness about your relationship to food.

Phase Two consists of a week of preparation before beginning the Very Low Calorie Diet. During this week, you are instructed on how to prepare your home by removing tempting foods, etc.. Attempts are made to include your family as a basic support system, and you are introduced to support group members and the behavioral group leader who is a psychologist.

Phase Three begins the liquid diet. During these two to 13 weeks, you completely replace solid food with the Optifast 70 or Optifast 800 Supplement taken five times per day. During this period, you visit with a physician every week, receive lab tests every two weeks to monitor physical condition, and attend a weekly group education session led by a team of health professionals such as registered dietitians, exercise specialists, and your behavioral group leader. Sessions focus on keeping on the supplement diet, developing a personalized and progressive exercise program, understanding the difference between physical and psychological hunger, dealing with stress, and nutritional education.

Phase Four runs seven weeks and is the period in which solid food is gradually reintroduced. First you are reintroduced to lean meats and vegetables while decreasing the Optifast supplements, and then proceed to the reintroduction of carbohydrates. During this period, you continue to see a physician every week and undergo laboratory tests every two weeks, and keep up your exercise program and weekly group sessions. The focus of the group now shifts to dealing with the reintroduction of food, how to successfully modify eating habits, how to identify relapses and minimize them, and specific lifestyle changes that can help keep the weight off.

Phase Five of the Optifast Program is the stabilization period and also lasts seven weeks. During this time, you are taken off Optifast Supplements completely and are instructed in a maintenance diet of food. You continue to have your health monitored through laboratory test every other week and continue weekly group meetings. The emphasis of the group sessions changes to issues pertaining to the new behavioral patterns necessary to maintaining weight loss, such as dealing with highly desired foods, identifying and handling high-risk situations, dealing with your emotions, and recovering from an overeating episode.

Phase Six is the Optifast "Encore Program" and lasts six months. It is designed to reinforce the new behavioral habits relative to diet and exercise so that you can successfully keep to a healthy weight. Group meetings continue, but now on a biweekly schedule.

THE DIET: Optifast produces two different supplements, Optifast 70 and Optifast 800. Both supply all the U.S. Recommended Daily Allowances. Optifast 70, which is mixed with any non-caloric beverage such as water, mineral water, or diet soda, is taken five times per day and consists of 420 calories and approximately 69 percent protein, 29 percent complex carbohydrates and less than two percent fat. Optifast 800 provides 800 calories for the larger-framed individual and consists of 35 percent protein, 50 percent carbohydrates and 15 percent fat.

As the food replacement is gradually removed during the stabilization and maintenance phase of the program, you are instructed in proper food choices and menu selection. The amount of calories consumed per day will depend upon whether you need to continue to lose weight or need to find the appropriate calories intake to maintain your new weight.

SUPPLEMENTAL PRODUCTS: None.

STAFF: The staff of Optifast Programs includes physicians, nurses, registered dietitians, and psychologists.

COSTS: Between $2600 and $3000 for the six-month program. This is inclusive of all physician visits, counseling, education, and meal supplements. As with all programs that include meal replacement products, in comparing costs you should consider the amount of money saved by not purchasing food at the grocery store during the meal replacement phase of the program.

AVERAGE WEIGHT LOSS: Four to five pounds per week.

PERSONAL CONSIDERATIONS: Optifast is an intensive medical program designed for people that are seriously obese. While many weight loss programs will accept individuals who are only moderately overweight or weigh 20 percent over their ideal weight, Optifast is specifically designed for people 50 to 100 pounds overweight. It is a Very Low Calorie diet and you should read the chapter on the history and issues surrounding Very Low Calorie Diets, and consult your doctor before making a decision.

Like all Very Low Calorie Diets, this system has the built-in problem of trying to retrain people to have better shopping and eating habits while at the same time requiring that they not shop or eat anything but the formula provided. The program does provide group counseling; however, while there is support and some assistance for developing an exercise plan, you must still exercise on your own.

LOCATION: Available nationwide. Contact the Sandoz Nutrition Corporation, 5320 West 23rd St., Minneapolis, MN 55416 (619) 593 2228 or consult your Yellow Pages.

ToppMed Inc.

The ToppMed program grew out of the experience of Dr. Frank Toppo, a specialist in obesity who practiced at the Obesity Clinic of the University of California at Irvine for six years. He began the program in 1985 with a liquid meal replacement formula, ToppFast, available through a national system of distributors. ToppMed's most recent product, ToppKrisp, is a chewable crispies meal replacement formula. Dr. Toppo's book, *The ToppFast Diet Plan* (1984), delineates the program's philosophy and emphasizes the importance of proper food choices.

HOW IT WORKS: The program is built around the belief that while the traditional Very Low Calorie Diet (usually consisting of complete meal replacement with a liquid formula) can be very effective in taking pounds off, it has shown much less success in allowing people to keep those pounds off. The ToppMed system, therefore, was designed to build in some real food experience during the weight loss phase. So its products are designed to be partial meal replacements.

ToppMed products can be used in two different programs. For those whose personal physicians have recommended rapid weight loss, ToppMed products can be used as a five-serving-per-day complete meal replacement diet of approximately 600 calories. (ToppMed advises that such a diet should only be undertaken with close monitoring from your doctor and will provide a complete "Physician Protocol" for your doctor's assistance.)

The regular program involves using ToppMed meal replacement products four times per day and eating one well-balanced, moderate calorie grocery store meal for a total diet of between 800 and 1000 calories per day. The program also provides weekly "ToppSupport" group meetings, and advises clients to begin an exercise program. ToppMed recommends that all potential users of its products consult their personal physician before starting any weight loss program.

THE DIET: This consists of four servings per day of either the ToppFast drink (vanilla and chocolate flavors), ToppFast chicken soup, or ToppKrisp crispies (Apple/Cinnamon, Nacho, and Chocolate flavors). The meal replacement formulas are interchangeable, so you can decide at any time which you'd prefer. Each serving of ToppFast formula is equal to 20 percent of the U.S. RDA. You also eat one well-balanced, moderate calorie regular meal per day for a total daily caloric intake of approximately 800 to 1000 calories. The program also recommends that you drink at least eight glasses of water per day.

SUPPLEMENTAL PRODUCTS: ToppMed produces a number of related products including chewable appetite control tablets, a nutritional supplement to increase short-term strength, and an isotonic carbohydrate and electrolyte replacement drink.

STAFF: Distributors also act as group leaders for ToppSupport meetings. They are trained by ToppMed and have access to the medical staff for answers to questions.

COST: ToppFast drinks are approximately $1.40 per serving (sold in 21-serving containers). ToppKrisp crispies are approximately $1.50 per serving.

AVERAGE WEIGHT LOSS: Depends on use. Suggested usage would result in one to two pounds per week. If used as a Very Low Calorie Diet under a physician's control, weight loss could be four to five pounds per week.

PERSONAL CONSIDERATIONS: Like other programs marketed through independent distributors, ToppMed requires a considerable degree of self-motivation and discipline. Your ToppMed distributor provides you with the products and will also arrange for some group support, but you have to take the lion's share of responsibility for directing your diet. For some this might be perfect; for others it might not work at all.

The ToppMed system has the benefit of requiring you to begin learning better grocery store and kitchen behavior patterns as you lose weight. This hands-on practice at breaking old food habits and developing more healthy ones should help in the long run; however, since it is basically a self operated program it is possible that your retraining could be less than completely satisfactory.

This system includes a few crunchy chewable food replacement options in addition to the standard shakes. For people that can't imagine just drinking breakfast and lunch, this is an added benefit. The program does not, however, provide much in the way of directed exercise assistance nor does it offer much help in modifying food behavior.

LOCATION: Sold nationwide, but only through ToppMed distributors. Call (800) 544-8677 for information regarding the distributor nearest you. To contact headquarters, call or write 1 Corporate Park Suite #100, Irvine, CA 92714 (714) 752-7337.

Combination Programs

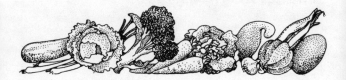

Cambridge/Food For Life

The Food For Life Weight Management System has its roots in a very low calorie supplement developed in 1970 by Alan Howard at the University of Cambridge in England. That program, based on a four-week cycle of replacing food with a very low calorie liquid formulation, was originally tested and marketed in Europe as the Cambridge Plan. It arrived in the United States in 1980, and reached its peak of popularity in 1981 and 1982; over five million individuals are estimated to have used the Cambridge Plan.

As the most visible of the first-generation liquid protein diets, the Cambridge Plan suffered from the fallout of criticism directed at a number of marginal liquid protein products. However, it now has been revived in a new, reformulated design, complete with a more comprehensive approach and a variety of different program options.

HOW IT WORKS: The Food For Life Weight Management System is available through Food For Life counselors and is designed to be self-guided with assistance from the counselor when and if necessary. The counselors are trained by the program to check to make sure that you don't have any health problems that would preclude participation in the program.

After meeting your counselor, you are briefed on the different program options. There are three: the Regular Program, the Fast-Start Program, and the Physician Monitored Program. Each is built around the Food For Life Ultimate Weight Loss Formula, which is a nutritious meal replacement formula available in a variety of drinks, soups, or flavored candy-style bars.

The Regular Program involves using the Food For Life Formula (drink, soup, or candy bar) three times a

97

day, and then eating an entree a day from the Food For Life Winning Food List. Since part of the program is an attempt to familiarize people with a wide variety of healthy foods, you are supposed to select a different entree every day for the first 21 days of the diet. Thereafter, and until you reach your goal weight, you can repeat entrees.

The Fast-Start Program is geared for losing ten to 15 pounds in two weeks for those who only need to lose that amount, as a way to get off to a quick start before going on the regular program, or to overcome plateaus encountered during the Regular Program. This method consists of a maximum two week period during which you consume three Food For Life Formula drinks, soups, or bars each day at regular meal times and control any hunger by snacking on extremely low calorie foods on the Food For Life's Free Food List.

The Physician Monitored Program is designed for individuals with 30 or more pounds to lose. It is similar to the Fast-Start Program in that Food For Life Formulas are consumed three times per day and the only solid food allowed is from the Free Food List. However, with the addition of close monitoring by a physician, you may continue the program beyond two weeks. Once your weight gets to within 15 pounds of your goal, you must shift over to the Regular Program and begin eating a selected entree from the Winning Foods List each day.

Each program is designed to be used in conjunction with a behavior modification system called Control For Life Learning Program, and an exercise program, Set For Life. Control For Life is a step by step self-instruction program designed to help you change undesirable eating habits; it includes two cassette tapes, one on behavioral modification and the other containing subliminal aids. It also comes with a workbook to help guide you through the dieting process, dealing with issues such as how to handle diet sabotage and how to relax.

The Set For Life Program is devised for people just beginning to exercise, and includes a walking program and a body conditioning and toning program. It comes with an elastic exercise aid device called the Set For Life Conditioner and Shaper, which is attached to a fixed object like a doorknob; the resistance it provides helps you to get the maximum benefit from exercise.

Additionally, your counselor is available to support your efforts by giving you information on recipes, maintaining weight records, and helping you to put together a personal support group.

The newest option offered by Food For Life is the Maintain For Life program. It consists of a 160 calorie drink that provides 100 percent of the U.S. Recommended Daily Allowances of all vitamins and minerals and 25 percent of required protein. It is designed to be used as an occasional one meal replacement in order to reduce calories and control appetite.

THE DIET: The heart of the diet is the Food For Life Ultimate Weight Loss Formula. The Formula is available as chocolate, vanilla, and strawberry drinks; chicken and tomato-flavored soup; and chocolate, coconut, and peanut candy-style bars. Taken three times per day, the Formula provides 100 percent of the U.S. Recommended Daily Allowance and equals approximately 400 calories, and is 44% protein, 53% carbohydrates and 3% fat.

During the Regular Program, the Formula is supplemented by one entree chosen from the Winning Food List. On the list are a wide variety of commercially available frozen entrees from Armour, Banquet Benihana, Chung King, Green Giant, Morton, and Stouffer's Lean Cuisine. Also included on the list are a number of recipes you can make yourself, such as Broiled Veal

Chops, Chicken Chow Mein Salad, Grilled Chicken with Wine, and Marinated Flank Steak.

SUPPLEMENTAL PRODUCTS: None.

STAFF: Food For Life is only available through counselors and distributors of the program. They are not health care professionals but are trained by the Program to teach the proper use of the program and to provide peer support.

COSTS: $120 covers the first month of food products plus the Control For Life and the Set For Life programs. Thereafter, food products run approximately $20 for a five-day supply.

AVERAGE WEIGHT LOSS: Regular Program: two to five pounds per week; Fast-Start Program or Physician Monitored Program: 16-20 pounds per month.

PERSONAL CONSIDERATIONS: The Food For Life Program involves a considerable amount of self-motivation and self-instruction. With a good counselor and a little luck, it is possible to receive group support, but it is not automatic. You should consider whether working toward your goal in more of a structured group setting would be best for you.

Also, while the weight loss formula is not cheap, you should remember when comparing costs that you are either not spending any money at the grocery store (in the case of the Fast-Start or the Physician Monitored programs) or at least are buying less at the store with the regular program. Of course, if you are not able to go without food, you may end up spending a lot more money—and gain weight, too.

The behavior modification and the exercise portions of the program are self-directed, and since both are vitally important to long term maintenance of weight loss, you should consider whether you will in fact diligently pursue them without outside encouragement.

Remember too, that the formula, when used under the Fast-Start or the Physician Monitored programs, qualifies under the definition of a Very Low Calorie Diet. You should read the chapter on Very Low Calorie Diets and consult your doctor before making a decision.

LOCATION: Available nationwide, but only through Food For Life Counselors or Distributors. Check your Yellow Pages under Weight Loss, or call 1-800-4-HEALTH for the name of a distributor near you. Headquarters are: Avadyne Incorporated, 2801 Salinas Highway, Monterey, CA 93940 (800) 443-2584.

Herbalife

Herbalife began in 1980 out of the trunk of Mark Hughes' car. His first product was a weight loss program that was marketed through word of mouth success stories, group meetings, and old-fashioned salesmanship. Contented customers became local distributors, and within ten years Herbalife had grown into one of the largest direct marketers of health care products in the world. Today Herbalife sells a variety of products including skin care and nutritional products in addition to its weight loss program.

HOW IT WORKS: The Herbalife plan is called the Diet Disc Program. It consists of drinking two Diet Disc Shakes per day, eating three Herbalife snacks per days, and having one regular meal.

Additionally, you are encouraged to take Herbalife vitamin-mineral tablets to assure you get adequate nutrition, and Herbalife Cell-U-Loss, a tablet product designed to assist elimination of excess fluids and reduce the appearance of cellulite.

Herbalife also suggests you take Activated Fiber

Tablets with meals to help create a feeling of fullness and Diet Disc Appezyme, a homeopathic compound to aid in appetite control.

Each Herbalife product includes a double-sided sheet of information of diet tips, a suggestion to supplement your diet with a moderate exercise regime, a chart for tracking weight loss, and recipes to go with Diet Disc beverages.

THE DIET: The diet consists of Diet Disc beverages (in French Vanilla, Dutch Chocolate, and Wild Berry), which, when combined with eight ounces of nonfat milk, equals approximately 175 calories per serving. The Diet Disc Shakes are used to replace two meals per day.

You are also allowed three snacks per day, chosen from Diet Disc Microwave Popcorn, or Raspberry or Cocoa Almond Nutrition Bars. The popcorn is 85 calories, the Raspberry Nutrition Bar is 90 calories and the Cocoa Almond Nutrition bar is 100 calories. You may also substitute some fresh fruit for one of the snacks.

For your one regular meal of the day, you are encouraged to select low fat, high fiber foods such as lean poultry, fish or meat, with fresh or steamed vegetables, a salad, and whole grains to equal between 350 and 500 calories total.

SUPPLEMENTAL PRODUCTS: Herbalife sells a wide variety of products through its independent distributors including nutritional products like mineral and vitamin supplements, a water treatment system, and skin care products for men and women.

STAFF: Herbalife is sold through independent distributors. Advice and assistance relative to the weight loss program will vary depending upon your distributor.

COST: The Diet Disc Program cost $100 and includes one container of Diet Disc Shakes, vitamin, fiber, and appetite control tablets, six nutrition bars (three of each flavor) and three packages of popcorn. This is enough for about a month.

AVERAGE WEIGHT LOSS: Approximately one to two pounds per week.

PERSONAL CONSIDERATIONS: Like many other programs marketed through independent distributors, this system requires a considerable degree of self-motivation and discipline. Your Herbalife distributor will make available all the products necessary for weight loss, and with luck you might get a distributor that is particularly helpful and encouraging, but basically you will have to direct your own diet. For some this might be ideal; for others it might well assure failure.

The Herbalife system does have the benefit of offering low-calorie snacks for the hopeless snackers among us. It doesn't provide much, however, in the way of directed exercise assistance nor does it offer much help in modifying your food behavior.

LOCATION: Herbalife is sold across the U.S., in Canada, Australia, England, Japan, and a number of other countries. Check the Yellow Pages or contact P.O. Box 80210, Los Angeles, CA 90009 (213) 410 9600.

Shaklee Corporation

The Shaklee Corporation was founded in 1956 by Dr. Forrest Shaklee, Sr. and has grown to one of the leading health corporations in the world. With a commitment to producing safe and environmentally sound products, the company offers a broad range of products from home cleaning solutions to water treatment systems, vitamins and mineral supplements, and a complete line of weight loss products.

HOW IT WORKS: Shaklee provides products and basic

information on suggested use through its system of independent distributors. You must do the rest yourself.

When purchasing diet products through a Shaklee distributor you also receive a brochure titled the "Shaklee Diet Guide" and a paper titled "The Physiology of Weight Loss." Combined, the information gives you a basic overview of the Shaklee program which is based on a meal replacement formula taken twice a day in addition to one well-balanced meal.

The program also includes taking a fiber supplement with every meal, fiber tablets between meals to help curb hunger, and a daily vitamin and mineral supplement. You are also encouraged to drink at least eight glasses of water per day and begin an exercise program to assist you in your weight loss efforts.

THE DIET: For two meals per day, instead of eating a regular meal, you either drink a Shaklee Slim Plan Beverage (Vanilla and Cocoa flavors) that is mixed with water, a Shaklee Meal Shake (French Vanilla and Bavarian Chocolate flavors) that is mixed with low-fat milk, or have a Slim Plan Cream of Chicken Soup or a Meal Soup Cream of Broccoli soup. Whichever you choose, you stir into it one tablespoon of Fiber Blend.

For the third meal of the day, you eat a balanced meal of one serving of protein, two servings of grains, two servings of fruit, two servings of fat (which can be replaced with increased servings from other food groups) and three servings of vegetables.

The Shaklee Diet Guide also provides a number of optional recipes as well as a list of healthy food choices in each of the food groups to select from for your regular meal of the day.

The Shaklee Slim Plan products contain 210 calories per serving and provide one third of the U.S. RDA; the Meal Shake and Meal Soup also provides one third of the RDA and contain 230 calories per serving.

SUPPLEMENTAL PRODUCTS: As mentioned above, Shaklee has a wide variety of health products from vitamin and mineral supplements to household products and personal care products.

STAFF: Not applicable.

COST: Meal Shakes cost approximately $16.80 per 15-serving container for approximately $1.05 per serving; Slim Plan Drink Mix run approximately $28.15 for 15 servings (around $1.90 per serving).

AVERAGE WEIGHT LOSS: Will depend on personal usage but if used according to the basic instructions approximately one to two pounds per week.

PERSONAL CONSIDERATIONS: This program is self-directed. One obvious requirement is the ability and motivation to discipline yourself. The program itself is relatively simple and has some of the benefits of any meal replacement program with the added benefit of daily training in good eating habits relative to planning your third meal of the day.

People who feel the need for more structure and support may not do well on this plan. And of course exercise is completely up to you. One final consideration is that the meal replacement formulas are not designed to be used as complete food replacements, and should not be used in that manner. See the chapter on Very Low Calorie Diets for more information and be sure to consult your own doctor.

WHERE LOCATED: Shaklee distributors can be found all across the U.S., in Puerto Rico, Canada, and Japan. Distributors can be found in the Yellow Pages or by calling 800-SHAKLEE. Corporate headquarters are at 444 Market Street, San Francisco, CA 94111 (800) 742 5533.

Slim Fast

Slim Fast products are purchased at retail outlets such as grocery stores. Each container includes a sheet with basic information on suggested product use. You can also write to the Slim Fast consumer department at the address given below and get additional recipes, menu suggestions, and nutritional and calorie information.

HOW IT WORKS: The Slim Fast program is based on a meal replacement formula taken twice a day combined with a well-balanced meal. Ultra Slim Fast is fortified with a natural fiber supplement to help curb hunger. The program also allows two snacks per day of fruit or vegetables if you feel the need. You are also encouraged to drink four or five glasses of water per day and begin an exercise program to assist you in your weight loss efforts.

The Slim Fast literature suggests that you can remain on this program for eight to 12 weeks and then shift to the maintenance plan. The maintenance plan simply replaces one of the Slim Fast drinks with another meal but allows for an additional Slim Fast drink as a snack.

THE DIET: For two meals per day, instead of eating a regular meal you either drink a Slim Fast or Ultra Slim Fast beverage (in vanilla, chocolate, and strawberry flavors) that is mixed with low-fat milk. For the third meal, you eat a regular well-balanced meal. The brochure that comes with containers of the product includes a number of meal suggestions.

Slim Fast contains 190 calories per serving and the Ultra Slim Fast contains 220 calories per serving. Both are formulated to provide one third of the U.S. RDA per serving. As long as you stick to the program and eat a moderate calorie meal for dinner, your daily caloric intake should be around 1100 to 1200 calories.

SUPPLEMENTARY PRODUCTS: Slim Fast also makes a peanut butter and a chocolate snack bar that is 140 calories each. When served with a six-ounce glass of skim milk, it totals 215 calories and can be used as a meal replacement instead of a drink.

COST: Slim Fast and Ultra Slim Fast are approximately $6 and $8 respectively per 13-serving container. Bars are approximately $4.99 to $5.99 for ten-bars boxes.

AVERAGE WEIGHT LOSS: This will depend on personal usage but if used according to the basic instructions approximately one to two pound per week.

PERSONAL CONSIDERATIONS: The Slim Fast Program is self directed. You purchase the products and get basic information on what to do, but the implementation is left up to you. One obvious requirement is the ability and motivation to discipline yourself. The program itself is relatively simple and has some of the benefits of any meal replacement program with the added benefit of daily training in good eating habits relative to planning your third meal of the day.

If you are looking to trim your weight without having to participate in a structured program or without having to be overly public about it, this kind of approach might be useful. On the other hand, those who feel the need for more structure and mutual support may not do all that well. Additionally, the sum total of the exercise component of this approach consists of a one paragraph note on the instruction sheet encouraging you to exercise.

One final consideration is that meal replacement formulas are not designed to be used as complete food replacements, and should not be used in that manner. See the chapter on Very Low Calorie Diets for more information, and be sure to consult your own doctor.

LOCATION: Slim Fast products can be found in most any grocery store, drug stores and frequently in retail discount centers. Manufactured by Thompson Medical Co. Inc., P.O. Box 5264, New York, New York 10150.

Other Weight Loss Programs

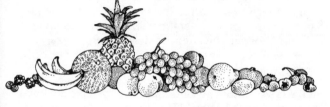

Larocque Diet Systems

Dr. Maurice Larocque (pronounced la-rock) is a highly respected physician in the field of obesity treatment who practices in Verdun, Quebec. After 20 years of research, he concluded that successful weight loss and particularly successful maintenance of weight loss, is more of a psychological problem than a physical one. Larocque believes that our attitudes, motivation, habits, self-image, and emotional responses determines what he calls our "mental weight." If, for example, our mental weight is 200 pounds, then dieting to 175 pounds will not help since in the long run we will simply return to our mental weight. To address this problem, Dr. Larocque has put together a program utilizing own computer software programs he affectionately calls Bert, Liza, and Adam, which are designed to help reduce a person's mental weight through mental exercises.

HOW IT WORKS: The Larocque Diet Systems are physician or hospital based. The system is unusual in a number of ways: it provides you with the option of different diet programs including the complete meal replacement regime of the Very Low Calorie Diets; one meal per day of grocery store food combined with meal replacement formulas for the other two meals; or a moderate calorie, grocery store food diet. It also makes extensive use of computer software, not only to design a diet regime tailored to the foods you prefer, but also to pinpoint possible psychological barriers to weight loss and to facilitate your interactive involvement in reducing your mental weight.

The program begins with a medical examination complete with EKG, assorted laboratory tests, and a body composition analysis. Then you and your physician determine what kind of diet you should be on and, with the help of Adam, the menu-planning software, you create a weekly diet plan meal by meal.

For the first two weeks of the program, you visit the center three days per week for what Larocque calls the "Fresh Start Phase." During this period you are introduced to the Larocque motivational library which includes four books titled *Be Thin Through Motivation, Be Thin, Master Your Emotions, Be Thin and Self-Confident,* and *Be Thin Day by Day*, two audio tapes, *Be Thin Be Motivated* and *Be Thin by Suggestion,* and two video tapes, *How to Overcome Guilt* and *How to Program Yourself Positively*.

During this period you are introduced to Bert and Liza. Bert is a computer program designed to assess your mental weight–the physical weight that you will keep returning to as long as the mental habits, behavior, and emotions revealed to Bert remain the same. You answer the questions Bert poses and Bert translates your responses by assigning a value to your attitudes and behaviors in regards to food. In addition, Bert will pinpoint problem areas that need "exercise" in order to reduce your mental weight, areas the staff will then help you resolve.

You also answer a series of questions posed by Liza, another software program. Liza's purpose is to uncover some of the root psychological issues that have helped program your current overweight condition so that they can be properly tended.

After the first two weeks you continue to visit the center on a weekly basis until you reach your goal weight for one on one assistance and physical monitoring. Individual counseling sessions emphasize working out problems that cause motivation blockage and developing good mental exercise habits. You then shift over to the maintenance program which lasts 12 months. Throughout this time you continue regular visits with Bert to monitor how your behavior and attitudes towards food is changing. Bert also flags particular problem areas and directs you to the appropriate video tape, audio tape, or book.

111

THE DIET: There is no single required diet with the Larocque System. After a consultation with your doctor you will jointly determine what kind of diet you should be on and what foods or nutritional formulas will be included. Options range from a strict Very Low Calorie Diet (see the chapter on Very Low Calorie Diets and consult your personal physician before choosing this option) where you forgo all grocery store food and replace it with Larocque's nutritional formula, to a moderate calorie diet (1200-1600 calories) that includes only grocery store food. You can also combine elements of both, by eating one meal per day of grocery store food and selecting supplement products for other meals and snacks.

SUPPLEMENTAL PRODUCTS: The Larocque system provides a wide variety of nutritional supplements including four flavors of shakes and puddings–Chocolate, Strawberry, Vanilla, and Banana, all 100 calories); three protein bars–Chocolate-Orange (140 calories), Honey-Peanut (140 calories) and Honey-Almond (130 calories); Hot Chocolate (80 calories); low calorie beverages in Orange, Lemon, Grape, and Grapefruit at 60 calories each; gelatin desserts in Strawberry and Lemon at 60 calories each; salad dressings in five flavors–French Style, Herb, Creamy Blue, Italian and Red Wine Vinegar–all at four calories per teaspoon; Chicken and Beef Bouillon, Cream of Chicken and Cream of Mushroom Soup at 70 calories each and Cream of Tomato, Cream of Onion and Cream of Asparagus Soup at 80 calories each.

STAFF: The Larocque System operates out of medical settings. Each program has at least one physician involved in medical monitoring and usually a nurse or other health care professional as well. Participating physicians and nurses are put through an extensive one-week certification training program and are regularly updated through bulletins and lectures.

COSTS: Cost will vary with location; however, the average program will cost around $440 including maintenance but excluding any food products. If you use the food supplements, they run approximately $10 per box which lasts around one week. It is an additional $149 for the Fresh Start package of four books, two audio tapes, and two video tapes.

AVERAGE WEIGHT LOSS: From two to five pounds per week depending upon diet.

PERSONAL CONSIDERATIONS: The Larocque system has a number of interesting features that make it different from much of the rest of the industry. Aside from the possible therapeutic value of the computer software, it may provide just the interactive computer fun necessary for some people to keep interested and motivated. Also, the concept of a "Mental Weight" is intriguing, although you should be aware that it not scientifically proven.

Additionally, the Larocque system offers a number of diet options that can be tailored to your specific needs, and offers a good deal more behavioral support than most other programs. However, it appears you are completely on your own as far as exercise is concerned, even though it is a crucial aspect of weight control.

LOCATION: The Larocque System has been available in Canada for many years, and is expanding rapidly in the United States. You can find the location nearest to you by calling or writing Great Health Inc., 4853 Medina Road, Akron, Ohio 44321 (800) 666-1717.

Overeaters Anonymous

Overeaters Anonymous (OA) began in Los Angeles in 1960 with three members who decided to create an organization patterned after the successful Alcoholics Anonymous to assist compulsive eaters in breaking their destructive habits. Like AA, there is a guarantee of confidentiality; there are no membership lists and registration is not required.

HOW IT WORKS: OA does not have weigh-ins, lectures, or diets. It is based on the premise that being overweight is only a symptom of the problem and that the compulsive eaters served by the organization use food in the same manner that alcoholics use alcohol.

OA members view their problem as physical, emotional, and spiritual. Those who attend meetings find a supportive group of admitted compulsive eaters who are committed to mutual support on the road to recovery. The OA philosophy has been adapted from the 12-step program used by Alcoholics Anonymous and includes the belief that assistance from God, as personally understood by each member, is essential to recovery.

OA believes that until compulsive eaters admit their problem they cannot solve it. So in practice the program begins with the admission that a person is a compulsive eater, obsessed with food, and that his or her own sheer will power is not enough. Dissatisfaction with weight alone, OA believes, will ultimately not be enough to allow full recovery. The battle begins with rigorous honesty and increased awareness of one's daily relationship to food.

THE DIET: OA does not advise regarding diets. They do, however, recommend that members strictly limit themselves to three moderate meals per day. Through this approach, compulsive eating habits hopefully can be brought under control.

SUPPLEMENTAL PRODUCTS: None.

STAFF: OA does not have a staff in any normal sense of the word. Local meetings are informal with some members taking responsibility for setting up locations, etc., but there is no hierarchy. The headquarters of OA acts to promote the awareness of the program, assures that adequate literature is available, and keeps in touch with local and regional groups.

COST: OA does not have any established fees. Costs of meeting places or any incidental expenses are covered by passing the hat. OA is committed to offering its service to anyone in need regardless of income.

AVERAGE WEIGHT LOSS: Not applicable.

PERSONAL CONSIDERATIONS: OA is set up to support people who admit they have a compulsive eating problem. So if you do not conceive of your weight problem in these terms, it probably won't work for you. Also, because one of the fundamental principles of OA involves the surrender of individual will to a higher power, anyone with a strong resistance to surrendering the concept of control may experience difficulty with the program.

LOCATION: Overeaters Anonymous is an international organization with meetings held in over 50 countries. Local information can be found through the World Service Center at P.O. Box 92870, Los Angeles CA 90009 or by calling (213) 542-8363.

Pritikin Longevity Centers

The Pritikin Longevity Centers grew out of Nathan Pritikin's 33-year battle against heart disease. After being diagnosed with coronary insufficiency in 1957, Pritikin developed his own comprehensive approach to health rooted in nutrition and exercise. While the program was originally designed for individuals with heart problems in mind, the overall program, focusing as it does on diet and exercise, is also used as an effective weight control program. The basics of the system are available in Robert Pritikin's book, *The New Pritikin Program* (1990).

HOW IT WORKS: The Pritikin Centers offer two residential programs. One is 13 weeks long and designed for those with a mild weight problem, hypertension, or mild diabetes. The second is 26 weeks and is primarily for people with advanced health problems such as heart disease or serious diabetes. The program runs throughout the year and involves a highly structured schedule of eating, exercise, and education.

Applicants are admitted only after they have sent their complete medical records to the Centers' medical offices in Santa Monica and have been approved. Upon arrival you are assigned to a physician appropriate to your condition (i.e., those with heart problems are assigned a cardiologist, etc.) and given a complete physical with blood tests; a medical history is also taken. You also have an in-depth discussion with your physician on the methods and goals of the program as it relates to you.

An exercise specialist then puts you through a treadmill tolerance test while monitoring an electrocardiogram in order to determine what kind and level of exercise program to place you in. You are then assigned to an exercise group supervised by the physiologist. This group includes exercise "classmates" who are at the same level of endurance, and with whom you will work out on a daily basis.

During your stay you meet regularly with a physician who monitors your progress, and keeps you informed of changing health indicators (e.g., if your blood pressure or cholesterol level is lowering, etc.). You also attend small classes dealing with issues pertinent to you such as workshops on weight control, stress management, lifestyle management, nutrition education, exercise, cooking classes, or other topics specific to differing health problems.

Here's an example of a typical day at the Center:

6:45: Wake-up and stretching exercises
7:30-9:30: Breakfast
8:00: Lecture (e.g., exercise and your heart)
9:10: Exercise class
9:30-10:30: Morning snacks
10:30: Doctor's appointment
11:00: Cooking class
11:30-2:30: Lunch
1:00: Lecture (e.g., composition of foods)
2:00: Exercise class
2:30-4:30: Afternoon snacks
3:00: Lecture (i.e. stress management)
4:00: Weight loss discussion
5:00: Walk, jog or run outdoors
6:00-7:15: Dinner
7:30: Entertainment

THE DIET: The Pritikin diet is composed of mainly fresh fruits and vegetables, whole grains such as brown rice and whole wheat bread, and other carbohydrates such as potatoes and pasta. No added sweeteners or fats are allowed. The nutritional breakdown of the diet is 75-80 percent complex carbohydrates, less than ten percent fat and ten to 15 percent protein. Unlike many diet programs, the Pritikin program does not rely on careful portion control. Most meals and snacks are served buffet style except for dinner, which is served by waitresses and waiters in the dining room.

SUPPLEMENTAL PRODUCTS: The Pritikin Center manufactures its own line of low fat food products that includes salad dressings, soups, sauces, pasta, snacks, spices, beverages, and entrees including frozen entrees. These products can be purchased at the Santa Monica store via telephone or mail.

STAFF: The staff at the Pritikin Longevity Centers includes medical doctors, licensed nurses, exercise specialists with either a B.A., B.S., or Master's degree in their specialty, registered dietitians, and licensed therapists.

COST: The standard fee for the 13-day program is $4509 and an optional $1406 for a spouse or companion. The 26-day program starts at $7614 with an optional $2711 for a spouse or companion. Fees are slightly higher for upgraded accommodations, and the Centers occasionally offer significant savings at specified times of the year.

AVERAGE WEIGHT LOSS: Thirteen pounds over four weeks for men, eight to 12 pounds over the same period for women. With continued use of the diet and exercise regime, you can expect approximately a one to two pound per week loss of weight.

PERSONAL CONSIDERATIONS: The Pritikin Longevity Centers are one of the more expensive weight loss options because they are residential programs. The residential aspect does have its advantages, however, in that it is both very intensive and highly structured. Under those circumstances the chances of relearning food behavior can be increased considerably. It also has the advantage of combining weight loss with a number of other concurrently running programs for people with heart disease and diabetes. Additionally, they emphasize a hands-on exercise program that can provide a great basis for after you return home.

One possible disadvantage is that once the residential program is over, you are pretty much on your own.

118

For those who can use the time during their stay to re-program their ideas and their behavior, that need not be a serious problem, but for people requiring ongoing support and guidance it could be a serious drawback. One possibility for those who need such assistance would be to join a support group type of program after returning home.

Another consideration is that during your residency at the Pritikin Center you are not shopping and cooking. This may be enough for some people to re-educate their palates (particularly those who always thought whole grains and vegetables were boring), but it might not be sufficient for others who may tend toward old habits when they get back into their own kitchens.

One final consideration is that the Pritikin diet is somewhat controversial in that it contains considerably less fat that is generally recommended (less than 10% of all calories coming from fat rather than 30%) and believe it or not, too little fat can cause its own problems. While many people would argue that given the ever presence of fat in American food products it is unlikely that many folks would end up suffering from too little fat, it is at least something you should be aware of.

LOCATION: Currently there are two Pritikin Longevity Centers–in Santa Monica, CA, and Miami Beach, FL. Contact the corporate headquarters at 1910 Ocean Front Walk, Santa Monica, CA 90405 (213) 450-5433 or (800) 421-9911 [(800) 421-0981 in CA].

TOPS Club, Inc.

TOPS, which stands for Take Pounds Off Sensibly, is the oldest weight loss organization in the country. It was founded in 1948 by Ester S. Manz who got together with a few overweight friends in Milwaukee and decided to apply the basic principles of Alcoholics Anonymous to weight loss. It currently has over 11,700 chapters in 19 countries. Unlike most weight loss programs, TOPS is a nonprofit, noncommercial organization.

HOW IT WORKS: The TOPS program is built around weekly, informal support meetings that operate on a completely democratic basis. Volunteer leaders are elected from the chapter membership, and discussions are directed and led by members with occasional guest speakers from health professionals. The emphasis of meetings is on mutual support and camaraderie--the program requires that your goal weight and diet plan be established by your personal physician.

TOPS also includes a strong emphasis on friendly competition with recognition for significant weight loss at local, state, and international levels, including the annual crowning of an international TOPS king and queen to the members who lost the most weight that year. Ongoing competition includes frequent recognition days. The club also has an inner honor society called KOPS (Keep Off Pounds Sensibly) for members who reach their goal weight and keep it off for at least 13 weeks.

TOPS also sponsors regular retreats that give members a chance to get out of their regular environment and combine a relaxing social event with an opportunity to pick up some information to help with weight loss.

Membership in TOPS includes a monthly edition of *TOPS News*, a magazine that provides running accounts of success stories, nutritional information, motivational features, low-calorie recipes, and news of chapter activities. In addition, TOPS annually contributes a portion of its income to an Obesity Research Program at the Medical College of Wisconsin.

THE DIET: TOPS publishes a nutritional monograph that it makes available to your doctor to explain its exchange system for planning meals and to assist the doctor in preparing a diet in consultation with you. But it prescribes no particular diet of its own.

SUPPLEMENTAL PRODUCTS: TOPS does not sell or endorse any products.

STAFF: Chapter meetings are organized by volunteer members who are assisted by a field staff of regional directors, coordinators, and area captains.

COST: Membership fees run $16 for the first two years in the U.S. and $14 each year thereafter ($20 and $18 respectively in Canada). There are no weekly fees.

AVERAGE WEIGHT LOSS: Not applicable.

PERSONAL CONSIDERATIONS: TOPS is a very informal organization that places heavy emphasis on mutual support and friendly competition. It is also one of the least expensive alternatives. If you are looking for group support to find your own way with a diet you and your doctor devise, and are motivated by competition, this may be the program for you. On the other hand, if you feel the need for a lot of pushing, prodding, one-on-one counseling, and over the shoulder monitoring in terms of food choices, behavior modification, and exercise, or if you hate competition, this may not be your best option.

LOCATION: Throughout the United States, Canada, and in 17 other countries. To find the group nearest you, check the Yellow Pages or contact International Headquarters, P.O. Box 07360, Milwaukee, WI 53207 (414) 482-4620.